Benyamin Schwarz
Editor

Assisted Living:
Sobering Realities

Assisted Living: Sobering Realities has been co-published simultaneously as *Journal of Housing for the Elderly*, Volume 15, Numbers 1/2 2001.

Pre-publication REVIEWS, COMMENTARIES, EVALUATIONS . . .

"A compilation of INSIGHTFUL, PENETRATING PERSPECTIVES: economic, social, historic, demographic, and personal. . . . Guides us in the evolution, maturation, and hope of assisted living. . . . A fitting tribute to the first editor and champion of *Housing for the Elderly*, Lee Pastalan."

Ruth Brent, PhD
Professor and Chair
Department of Environmental Design
University of Missouri, Columbia

Assisted Living: Sobering Realities

Assisted Living: Sobering Realities has been co-published simultaneously as *Journal of Housing for the Elderly*, Volume 15, Numbers 1/2 2001.

The *Journal of Housing for the Elderly* Monographic "Separates"

Below is a list of "separates," which in serials librarianship means a special issue simultaneously published as a special journal issue or double-issue *and* as a "separate" hardbound monograph. (This is a format which we also call a "DocuSerial.")

"Separates" are published because specialized libraries or professionals may wish to purchase a specific thematic issue by itself in a format which can be separately cataloged and shelved, as opposed to purchasing the journal on an on-going basis. Faculty members may also more easily consider a "separate" for classroom adoption.

"Separates" are carefully classified separately with the major book jobbers so that the journal tie-in can be noted on new book order slips to avoid duplicate purchasing.

You may wish to visit Haworth's website at . . .

http://www.HaworthPress.com

. . . to search our online catalog for complete tables of contents of these separates and related publications.

You may also call 1-800-HAWORTH (outside US/Canada: 607-722-5857), or Fax 1-800-895-0582 (outside US/Canada: 607-771-0012), or e-mail at:

getinfo@haworthpressinc.com

Assisted Living: Sobering Realities, edited by Benyamin Schwarz, PhD (Vol. 15, No. 1/2, 2001). *Explores the implications of the current state of one of the fastest-growing areas in housing for the elderly.*

Housing Choices and Well-Being of Older Adults: Proper Fit, edited by Leon A. Pastalan, PhD, and Benyamin Schwarz, PhD (Vol. 14, No. 1/2, 2001). *"Convincing . . . Helpful in improving accessibility. . . . With this collaborative work we are one step closer to taming fears, domesticating dreams, and realizing gerontopia." (Ruth S. Brent, PhD, Professor and Chair, Department of Environmental Design, University of Missouri-Columbia)*

Making Aging in Place Work, edited by Leon A. Pastalan, PhD (Vol. 13, No. 1/2, 1999). *Addressing issues ranging from home modification to treatment of depression, this book will help you identify the needs of the elderly in order to offer them a comfortable and more independent life.*

Shelter and Service Issues for Aging Populations: International Perspectives, edited by Leon A. Pastalan, PhD (Vol. 12, No. 1/2, 1997). *"Provides an international perspective on meeting the housing and service needs of the elderly. The book outlines the strengths and weaknesses of different approaches, policies, and cost-effective, successful arrangements." (Older Americans Report)*

Housing Decisions for the Elderly: To Move or Not to Move, edited by Leon Pastalan, PhD (Vol. 11, No. 2, 1995). *"This insightful book thoroughly explores the crucial decisions many elderly face, and it provides a comprehensive overview of the complex problems that are associated with these decisions." (Benyamin Schwarz, PhD, Assistant Professor, Environmental Design Department, University of Missouri)*

University-Linked Retirement Communities: Student Visions of Eldercare, edited by Leon A. Pastalan, PhD, and Benyamin Schwarz (Vol. 11, No. 1, 1994). *"A masterpiece. . . . Provides one of the most comprehensive sets of illustrations for integrating research-based theory with design to date. . . . The contribution this book makes to a better understanding of the multidisciplinary nature of the design process is profound."(Ronald G. Phillips, ArchD, Director, Graduate Studies Program, Department of Environmental Design, University of Missouri-Columbia)*

Congregate Housing for the Elderly: Theoretical, Policy, and Programmatic Perspectives, edited by Lenard W. Kaye, DSW, and Abraham Monk, PhD (Vol. 9, No. 1/2, 1992). *"Significant authorities present concise factual chapters about federal housing policies, services for elders, models of service assisted housing, enhanced or supported housing and 'assisted living,' and* *specifically, the federal congregate Housing Services Program." (Journal of the American Geriatrics Society)*

Residential Care Services for the Elderly: Business Guide for Home-Based Eldercare, edited by Doris K. Williams, PhD (Vol. 8, No. 2, 1991). *"A how-to-do-it manual for persons considering establishing a home-based business to provide residential care services for elderly people." (Science Books & Films)*

Housing Risks and Homelessness Among the Urban Elderly, edited by Sharon M. Keigher, PhD (Vol. 8, No. 1, 1991). *"A good beginning for an understanding of homelessness among older persons. . . . Useful for policymakers in their pursuit of useful and valid information that would serve to focus the direction of future policies and programs related to homelessness, especially among those who are older." (Educational Gerontology)*

Granny Flats as Housing for the Elderly: International Perspectives, edited by N. Michael Lazarowich, PhD (Vol. 7, No. 2, 1991). *"An informative guide to the latest experimental projects and government programs to encourage the provision of 'granny flats' or 'echo housing'-apartment or other dwelling units which are wholly or partly linked to or within a family dwelling." (Tony Warnes, Kings College, London)*

Optimizing Housing for the Elderly: Homes Not Houses, edited by Leon A. Pastalan, PhD (Vol. 7, No. 1, 1991). *"Especially helpful to planners and policy developers in the area of housing alternatives for the elderly. There is a clear effort to provide a range of options for professional intervention." (Science Books & Films)*

Aging in Place: The Role of Housing and Social Supports, edited by Leon A. Pastalan, PhD (Vol. 6, No. 1/2, 1990). *"Emphasizes the practicalities of keeping people going in independent housing." (British Journal of Psychiatry)*

The Retirement Community Movement: Some Contemporary Issues, edited by Leon Pastalan, PhD (Vol. 5, No. 2, 1989). *The practical implications of the research findings provided in this key volume help readers to identify and satisfy the needs of retirement community residents.*

Lifestyles and Housing of Older Adults: The Florida Experience, edited by Leon A. Pastalan, PhD, and Marie E. Cowart, DPH, RN (Vol. 5, No. 1, 1989). *"A good introductory source for students to understand recent efforts to amalgamate living environments and service delivery systems in order to provide better care for the elderly." (Community Alternatives)*

Aging at Home: How the Elderly Adjust Their Housing Without Moving, edited by Raymond J. Struyk, PhD, and Harold M. Katsura, MCRP (Vol. 4, No. 2, 1988). *"Of value in the development of a comprehensive theory of environmental adjustment relevant regardless of age for those for whom living in place has become problematic." (Disabilities Studies Quarterly)*

Continuing Care Retirement Communities: Political, Social, and Financial Issues, edited by Ian A. Morrison, Ruth Bennett, PhD, Susana Frisch, MA, and Barry J. Gurland, MD (Vol. 3, No. 1/2, 1986). *"Well-written and comprehensive in scope." (The Gerontologist)*

Retirement Communities: An American Original, edited by Michael E. Hunt, Allan G. Feldt, Robert W. Marans, Leon A. Pastalan, and Kathleen L. Vakalo (Vol. 1, No. 3/4, 1984). *A thorough, informative volume on retirement communities in the United States.*

Assisted Living: Sobering Realities

Benyamin Schwarz
Editor

Assisted Living: Sobering Realities has been co-published simultaneously as *Journal of Housing for the Elderly,* Volume 15, Numbers 1/2 2001.

The Haworth Press, Inc.
New York • London • Oxford

Assisted Living: Sobering Realities has been co-published simultaneously as *Journal of Housing for the Elderly*™, Volume 15, Numbers 1/2 2001.

The Haworth Press, Inc., 10 Alice Street, Binghamton, NY 13904-1580

Cover Design by So-Yeon Yoon

Library of Congress Cataloging-in-Publication Data

Assisted living: sobering realities/Benyamin Schwarz, editor.
  p. cm.
  ". . . has been co-published simultaneously as Journal of housing for the elderly, volume 15, numbers 1/2 2001."
  Includes bibliographical references and index.
  ISBN 0-7890-1443-2 (hardback: alk. paper)--ISBN 0-7890-1444-0 (soft: alk. paper)
  1. Aged--Housing. I. Schwarz, Benyamin. II. Journal of housing for the elderly.

HD7287.9 .A87 2001
362.1'16'0973 –dc21

2001039662

Indexing, Abstracting & Website/Internet Coverage

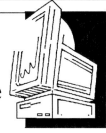

This section provides you with a list of major indexing & abstracting services. That is to say, each service began covering this periodical during the year noted in the right column. Most Websites which are listed below have indicated that they will either post, disseminate, compile, archive, cite or alert their own Website users with research-based content from this work. (This list is as current as the copyright date of this publication.)

Abstracting, Website/Indexing Coverage . . . . Year When Coverage Began

- *Abstracts in Social Gerontology: Current Literature on Aging* **1992**

- *AgeInfo CD-ROM* **1997**

- *AgeLine Database* **1994**

- *AGRICOLA Database* **1992**

- *Applied Social Sciences Index & Abstracts (ASSIA) (Online: ASSI via Data-Star) (CDRom: ASSIA Plus) <www.bowker-saur.co.uk>* **1992**

- *Architectural Periodicals Index* **1992**

- *CINAHL (Cumulative Index to Nursing & Allied Health Literature), in print, EBSCO, and SilverPlatter, Data-Star, and PaperChase. (Support materials include Subject Heading List, Database Search Guide, and instructional video.)* **1997**

- *CNPIEC Reference Guide: Chinese National Directory of Foreign Periodicals* **1997**

- *Family & Society Studies Worldwide <www.nisc.com>* **1997**

- *FINDEX <www.publist.com>* **1999**

(continued)

Special Bibliographic Notes related to special journal issues (separates) and indexing/abstracting:

- indexing/abstracting services in this list will also cover material in any "separate" that is co-published simultaneously with Haworth's special thematic journal issue or DocuSerial. Indexing/abstracting usually covers material at the article/chapter level.
- monographic co-editions are intended for either non-subscribers or libraries which intend to purchase a second copy for their circulating collections.
- monographic co-editions are reported to all jobbers/wholesalers/approval plans. The source journal is listed as the "series" to assist the prevention of duplicate purchasing in the same manner utilized for books-in-series.
- to facilitate user/access services all indexing/abstracting services are encouraged to utilize the co-indexing entry note indicated at the bottom of the first page of each article/chapter/contribution.
- this is intended to assist a library user of any reference tool (whether print, electronic, online, or CD-ROM) to locate the monographic version if the library has purchased this version but not a subscription to the source journal.
- individual articles/chapters in any Haworth publication are also available through the Haworth Document Delivery Service (HDDS).

Assisted Living:
Sobering Realities

CONTENTS

ABOUT THE EDITOR

Benyamin Schwarz, PhD, is Associate Professor in the Department of Environmental Design at the University of Missouri-Columbia. He received his bachelor's degree in Architecture and Urban Planning from the Technion, the Institute of Technology of Israel, and his PhD in Architecture with an emphasis on Environmental Gerontology from the University of Michigan. He designed numerous projects in Israel and consulted with many retirement communities in the U.S. His teaching specialty areas include design fundamentals, housing concepts and issues, design studio, architectural programming, and environmental design for aging. His research addresses issues of long-term care settings in the United States and abroad, environmental attributes of dementia special care units, assisted living arrangements, and international housing concepts and issues. Dr. Schwarz is the author of *Nursing Home Design: Consequences of Employing the Medical Model* (Garland Publishing, Inc., 1996). He co-edited, with Leon A. Pastalan, *University-Linked Retirement Communities: Student Visions of Eldercare* (The Haworth Press, Inc., 1994) and *Housing Choices and Well-Being of Older Adults: Proper Fit* (The Haworth Press, Inc., 2001). He co-edited, with Ruth Brent, *Aging, Autonomy, and Architecture: Advances in Assisted-Living* (The Johns Hopkins University Press, 1999) and *Popular American Housing: A Reference Guide* (Greenwood Press, 1995).

Introduction

Benyamin Schwarz

Assisted living is arguably the most significant development in the field of planned housing and services for older adults in the U.S. in recent years. According to one source, this type of senior housing provides shelter and care services for an estimated one million individuals in 30,000-40,000 facilities (PricewaterhouseCoopers, 1998). While definitions may vary considerably, assisted living is "a long-term care alternative that involves the delivery of professionally managed personal and health care services in a group setting that is residential in character and appearance; it has the capacity to meet unscheduled needs for assistance, while optimizing residents' physical and psychological independence" (Regnier, 1999:3).

While the emergence of assisted living is a relatively recent phenomenon, various housing models that respond to the needs of frail older persons who do not wish or cannot manage to live alone, or who no longer can handle the challenges of their home environment, have been available for a long time. The philosophy that separates assisted living from other housing models with varying levels of oversight and care provides residents with the chance to avoid institutionalization and maintain their remaining functional independence in a residential environment. In an ideal world, assisted living is a model of long-term care that offers frail elders a broad set of choices by separating the "nursing" component from the room-and-board component.

The primary goal of assisted living is to provide services tailored to individual needs in a residential and normalized setting. The care and aid options may include meals, assistance with housekeeping, laundry, and bathing as well as personal and functional support services related to activities of daily living. While many facilities are not prepared to provide long-term medical care, most of them have 24-hour emergency response programs on-site. These essential services are

[Haworth co-indexing entry note]: "Introduction." Schwarz, Benyamin. Co-published simultaneously in *Journal of Housing for the Elderly* (The Haworth Press, Inc.) Vol. 15, No. 1/2, 2001, pp. 1-4; and: *Assisted Living: Sobering Realities* (ed: Benyamin Schwarz) The Haworth Press, Inc., 2001, pp. 1-4. Single or multiple copies of this article are available for a fee from The Haworth Document Delivery Service [1-800-342-9678, 9:00 a.m. - 5:00 p.m. (EST). E-mail address: getinfo@haworthpressinc.com].

typically provided in self-contained private apartments, each with a kitchen, bathroom, and sleeping and living areas. Frequently, the facilities consist of a small cluster of apartments with shared, public areas. Design features such as lockable doors, individual temperature controls, communication systems, and personal furniture and accessories are widespread attributes in these settings.

Several states have allowed the development of assisted-living arrangements in the last decade, in response to both consumer demand and dwindling federal and state resources. Nevertheless, such long-term care options are still more likely to be available to middle- and upper-income elders who can afford to pay privately for these services. Regrettably, the combined characteristics of lower income and frailty tend to lead people to subsidized housing, in which professional nursing or therapy are not provided, or to medically oriented long-term care institutions (Schwarz & Brent, 1999).

As more assisted-living facilities are maturing, some sobering realities are emerging and research into the field is growing. Two symposia sponsored by the International Assisted Living Foundation of America (IALF) were presented in November 2000 during the annual meeting of the Gerontological Society of America (GSA) in Washington, D.C. The presentations highlighted research findings in ten different areas, addressing practices, policies, and outcomes across multiple assisted living settings. In addition, findings related to aging-in-place, social function and service provision, end-of-life care, determinants of medical outcomes, and comparisons of outcomes for persons with dementia in assisted living and nursing homes were discussed.

The IALF was founded by the Assisted Living Federation of America (ALFA) to support consumer education, research, and global issues to benefit persons affected by the assisted-living industry. An Assisted Living Interest Group composed of long-term care researchers, practitioners, health and aging managers, policy makers, directors, and community and product developers and marketers was recently established by members of the Gerontological Society of America (GSA). This group plans to meet at least annually at the GSA to promote the conduct of interdisciplinary research in assisted living that is guided by the needs of providers, consumers, and policy makers; to expand the quantity and improve the quality of research related to assisted living; to increase the funding resources available to pursue research in assisted living; and to establish and further mechanisms whereby findings related to assisted living are brought to the attention of policy makers and practitioners.

One notable program of assisted-living research is known as the Collaborative Studies of Long-Term Care, being conducted by the Cecil G. Sheps Center for Health Services Research, University of North Carolina at Chapel Hill, by Drs. Sheryl Zimmerman, Philip Sloane, and Kevin Eckert. These studies are being conducted in almost 250 residential care, assisted-living facilities, and nursing homes across four states, and include all types of facilities, ranging from small "mom and pop" homes to new-model assisted living. The goals of the collaborative studies are to further the quality of life and quality of care of residents, including consideration of families and long-term care workers. Funding sources for the program include the National Institute on Aging; the Alzheimer's Association, the Retirement Research Foundation, and the Mather Foundation (Zimmerman, 2000).

Some of the recent research and thinking on a range of important topics pertaining to assisted living have been included in this collection. Jacquelyn Frank commences with findings from her anthropological fieldwork in two assisted living sites in Chicago, Illinois, in which she discusses the fundamental question of aging-in-place in assisted-living settings from providers and residents' perspectives. The reader is then presented with findings from a study reported by Thompson, Weber, and Juozapavicius that sought to explore the influence of visitation patterns on the life satisfaction of residents in five assisted-living facilities in Oklahoma. Damron-Rodriguez, Harada, and McGuire proceed to examine characteristics of 109 residents in two Residential Care Facilities for the Elderly (RCFEs) in Los Angeles, California, in an attempt to understand the role of RCFEs in community-based long-term care. Newcomer, Swan, and Karon subsequently present their findings from a study of state policies affecting nursing homes and residential care facilities in Kansas, Maine, Mississippi, Ohio, and South Dakota. Crook and Vinton then present their survey of 140 assisted-living facilities in Florida that was designed to solicit information about the organizational characteristics of these housing and services arrangements. The discussion about assisted living concludes with Marsden's chapter, which outlines the concept of *home* and the search for transferable residential attributes that symbolize the home environment in the design of housing for the elderly.

The subsequent chapters bring to the fore topics regarding accommodations for low-income older adults. Cox reports on a study that compared facilities from the 1994 HUD's Best Practice competition in an attempt to demonstrate how winning facilities established more effective approaches to comprehensive service provision, provided wider range of health and social services, and were more successful in linking low-income elders with community-based services. Finally, Bogdon, Katsura, and Mikelsons review different measures of poverty and housing problems to reveal unmet needs of housing assistance for elderly people.

This set of articles addresses some of the sobering realities and raises issues for those engaged in shaping the future of assisted living.

REFERENCES

PricewaterhouseCoopers. 1998. *An Overview of the Assisted Living Industry*, 1998. Fairfax, VA: Assisted Living Federation of America.

Regnier, V. 1999. The definition and evolution of assisted living within a changing system of long-term care. In B. Schwarz and R. Brent, eds., *Aging Autonomy and Architecture: Advances in Assisted Living*. Baltimore, MD: The Johns Hopkins University Press.

Schwarz, B., and R. Brent, Eds. 1999. *Aging Autonomy and Architecture: Advances in Assisted Living*. Baltimore, MD: The Johns Hopkins University Press.

Zimmerman, S. [Sheryl_Zimmerman@unc.edu] (2000, November 26). Personal e-mail.

Chapter 1

How Long Can I Stay?: The Dilemma of Aging in Place in Assisted Living

Jacquelyn Frank

SUMMARY. Aging in place has long been a focus for proponents of assisted living housing. However, the reality of life for seniors in assisted living is often tenuous, and this homelike setting repeatedly ends up being a temporary stop for older adults. Residents frequently ask, "How long can I stay?", only to find that there is no easy answer. Increasing frailty and declining health can mean that an elderly resident may be asked to leave assisted living, reducing aging in place in this housing/health care option to what I have termed "prolonged residence."

Based on eighteen months of anthropological fieldwork at two assisted living sites in Chicago, Illinois, this article presents the individual struggles providers and residents face in interpreting aging in place. Although grappling with disparate aspects of the same issue, residents and providers both share conflicted feelings about how long one should remain in assisted living and what aging in place actually means. *[Article copies available for a fee from The Haworth Document Delivery Service: 1-800-342-9678. E-mail address: <getinfo@haworthpressinc.com> Website: <http://www.HaworthPress.com> © 2001 by The Haworth Press, Inc. All rights reserved.]*

KEYWORDS. Assisted living, aging in place, residents' realities, providers' views, prolonged residence, liminality

Jacquelyn Frank, PhD, is Assistant Professor and Coordinator of Gerontology Programs, Department of Sociology-Anthropology, Illinois State University, Campus Box 4660, Normal, IL 61790-4660.

[Haworth co-indexing entry note]: "Chapter 1. *How Long Can I Stay?*: The Dilemma of Aging in Place in Assisted Living." Frank, Jacquelyn. Co-published simultaneously in *Journal of Housing for the Elderly* (The Haworth Press, Inc.) Vol. 15, No. 1/2, 2001, pp. 5-30; and: *Assisted Living: Sobering Realities* (ed: Benyamin Schwarz) The Haworth Press, Inc., 2001, pp. 5-30. Single or multiple copies of this article are available for a fee from The Haworth Document Delivery Service [1-800-342-9678, 9:00 a.m. - 5:00 p.m. (EST). E-mail address: getinfo@haworthpressinc.com].

INTRODUCTION

Currently, aging in place is a subject of much discussion and debate among assisted living providers, designers, researchers, and policy-makers (Mollica et al. 1995; Heumann and Boldy 1993a; Pynoos 1990; Sherwood et al. 1990; Callahan 1993). Questions such as who qualifies as an appropriate candidate for assisted living and how long a resident may stay are becoming more complicated with the expansion of this supportive housing option. Should assisted living remain part of the conventional continuum of care or should residents truly be allowed to age in place until they die, regardless of their level of impairment (Wilson 1990)? These questions are of concern not only to researchers, but especially to providers and residents who must face these dilemmas daily in assisted-living communities.

This article focuses on the experiences of residents and providers at several assisted-living sites in Chicago, Illinois. Specifically, questions are raised regarding how providers and residents interpret aging in place and what repercussions these interpretations have on assisted-living policies. The article begins by focusing on the variety of present assisted-living models across the country. Highlighted are the types of services and physical environments offered by each model. Following this, I discuss the variety of interpretations for the phrase "aging in place." Next, the focus shifts to providers and their explanation of aging in place as it applies to their individual facility policies. Admission and discharge criteria are examined at several assisted living facilities in order to illustrate the complexity of the aging in place issue. Revealed is the fact that most providers interpret aging in place to mean what I have termed *"prolonged residence."* Prolonged residence only allows residents of assisted living to stay for an undetermined, vague period of time that is never made clear to the resident.

Next, the viewpoints of residents are examined. How do older adults in assisted living reconcile the tension between their own desire to age in place but not live among an impaired population? The research method used in this project allowed both providers and residents to offer their personal feelings and attitudes on assisted living. Presenting the residents' and providers' own words in the article reveals the emotional nature of the aging in place debate. Finally, these various interpretations of aging in place are analyzed in relation to prolonged residence and the goals and principles of assisted living housing.

Exactly what assisted living *is* remains a question that is answered by individual states and facilities (Mollica et al. 1992). It should be noted here that the ambiguity surrounding a universal definition of assisted living creates both great flexibility and great confusion for providers as well as consumers. Ambiguity allows providers to develop policies and rules specifically geared toward their particular facility or state requirements. At the same time, without a standard definition of assisted living, policy decisions such as entrance and discharge criteria are more difficult for providers and more stressful for residents.

There is general consensus, however, regarding the philosophy of care that surrounds assisted living. Scholars agree that the basic philosophy of assisted living includes maximizing privacy, dignity, independence, choice, and autonomy for residents (Regnier et al. 1991; Kane and Wilson 1993; Kalymun 1990; ALFA 1994). This is accomplished through the creation of a homelike environment and supportive services. Exactly *how* this is carried out varies from one assisted living community to the next.

The data for this article was gathered during eighteen months of research in the Chicago, Illinois, metropolitan area. Two primary assisted living sites were utilized to gather qualitative data. The first facility, *Kramer*, is a free-standing site housing twenty-nine residents in suburban Chicago. The second site, *The Wood Glen Home*, is actually a nursing home containing one floor devoted to assisted living.[1] *The Wood Glen Home* is located in the city of Chicago, and its assisted-living unit houses up to eighteen people. Participant-observation fieldwork was conducted for a year and a half at both sites. The research consisted of multiple tape-recorded interviews with residents and providers, informal interviews and discussions, participation in resident activities, and the administration of anonymous surveys.[2] I also visited eight other assisted living sites in the Chicago area and conducted interviews with administrators at each facility. Through daily interaction, in-depth interviews, and anthropological analysis, it is clear that providers and residents are both concerned with the future of aging in place in assisted living.

ASSISTED LIVING: EVOLUTION AND MODELS

Assisted living refers to a housing/health care alternative for elderly persons who are no longer able to live independently in their own homes but do not require 24 hour nursing care (Regnier 1991). A unique dimension of assisted living is the fact that there is no one standard definition for this residential option. The Assisted Living Federation of America (ALFA), the American Association of Homes and Services for the Aging (AAHSA), the U.S. Health Care Financing Administration (HCFA), as well as various scholars, such as Regnier (1996), Mollica and Snow (1996), and Wilson (1996), have all posed definitions of assisted living. Although the definitions may differ, there are two components present in virtually all definitions. These two commonalties include assisted living as a combination of some kind of housing *and* services. This is where the similarities usually end. Individual states will then decide what is meant by "housing" and what is meant by "services" for their definitions, policies, and procedures.

In order to clarify some of the confusion, ALFA (1999) has offered two general models of assisted living. The first type of assisted living is referred to as the "Senior Housing with Non-Health Care Services" model. Services that are generally provided in this model of assisted living are non-medical in nature and include meals, housekeeping, transportation, security, and very limited personal assistance with activities of daily living (ADLs). "It focuses on maintaining a strong residential characteristic with little emphasis on health services" (ALFA 1999:7). In other words, services focus on Instrumental Activities of Daily Living (IADLs). The major limitations of the model are that personal care is minimal and nursing care is nonexistent, often resulting in shorter residency for older adults and a high turnover for the assisted living community. This model also poses serious barriers to aging in place because there is no assistance present to help a resident who experiences increasing frailty or health complications.

The Assisted Living Federation of America (ALFA) offers a second model of assisted living called "Senior Housing with Health Care Services." Residences under this model provide meals, transportation, housekeeping, and security as in the first model. However, this plan also includes significant personal assistance, health monitoring, and often 24-hour on-site nursing staff, and nursing services. One feature of this model is that it offers specialized assisted living communities for people with Alzheimer's disease. "This model focuses on health services and the concept of *aging in place*" (ALFA 1999:8). The benefits of this model are that it allows for the possibility of aging in place and results in a lower rate of resident turnover. The major roadblock for this model is licensing. "Even the inclusion of minor health services may trigger a requirement that the facility get licensed" (ibid.). Licensure can result for a provider if the setting supplies services that meet the definition of a licensed level of care for that state, whether or not it is called assisted living.

In a separate work, Hawes (1999) proposes a more detailed division of assisted living models. Based on a national study of 11,500 assisted living sites in the United States, she found that there are four basic types of assisted living that are represented across the country. Although not related to the models proposed by ALFA, Hawes' four categories fit nicely into the two classifications discussed above.

The first type described by Hawes is termed "Low Service/Low Privacy." Nationwide, this form represents 59% of the places that call themselves assisted living. In the low service/low privacy model, the majority of rooms are shared and offer ADL assistance only with bathing and dressing. Most of the services provided here would be for IADLs.

The second type of assisted living community Hawes refers to as "Low Service/High Privacy." Approximately 18% of the 11,500 assisted living sites in the United States represent this model. Here, residents would likely have a private room (or apartment) and a private bathroom but not much in the way of ADL assistance. Hawes has also referred to this model as the "cruise ship" model because of its emphasis on luxury, privacy, and hospitality services. Of my two research sites, Kramer's assisted living community would fit into this category.

The third type of assisted living described by Hawes is "High Service/Low Privacy." In these assisted living settings, two-thirds of residents live in rooms rather than apartments, and slightly over 20% of the rooms are shared. All of the high service/low privacy sites in Hawes' study had an RN on staff, and the respondents for these sites all claimed that they would retain a resident who needed nursing care. Nationally, only 12% of assisted living communities fall into this category. Assisted living at Wood Glen conforms to the High Service/Low Privacy category.

The final model Hawes presents is called the "High Service/High Privacy" model. This group offers both private dwellings for residents as well as a high level of services to meet both ADL and IADL needs. Approximately 11% of assisted living sites nationwide qualify for this category.

The Low Service/Low Privacy model and the Low Service/High Privacy model both conform to the first ALFA category above, Senior Housing with Non-Health Care Services. Hawes' two models could be seen as a subcategory of the ALFA classification because both of these models have a lower emphasis on services, and virtually no emphasis on health-related care. The High Service/Low Privacy and the High Service/High Privacy models qualify under the second ALFA model because both are geared toward meeting the health needs of residents. This second set of models offers a greater possibility of aging in place because they can supply the needed health care and advanced ADL assistance that a resident may need to remain in assisted living. However, even the high service models do not guarantee that residents will be permitted to fully age in place.

The distinctions between these four models are critical to detail because several of the models Hawes presents do not adhere to the basic philosophy of care that is so central to assisted living. "Assisted living's philosophy is to provide physically and cognitively impaired older persons the personal and health-related services that they require to age in place in a homelike environment that maximizes their dignity, privacy, independence, and autonomy" (Wilson 1996:10). Three of the four assisted living models outlined above would not qualify as complying with the philosophy of care stated by Wilson, and would therefore lack the essence of what assisted living strives to be. Presently, it will be useful to flesh out the various meanings of aging in place in order to provide a framework for providers' and residents' experiences in assisted living.

WHAT DOES IT MEAN TO AGE IN PLACE?

Aging in place is defined in the *Dictionary of Gerontology* as "the effect of time on a non-mobile population; remaining in the same residence where one has spent his or her earlier years" (Harris 1988:18). This strict definition of aging in place refers only to changes that occur to the occupants over time; it does not address the changing nature of the environment itself. In fact, several definitions of aging in place offered by scholars in recent years focus almost exclusively on changes in the inhabitants, overlooking changes in the environment (Mangum 1994; Callahan 1993; Merrill and Hunt 1990). Nevertheless, housing is not static.

In contrast to these narrow definitions, Lawton (1990) describes aging in place as a much more multi-dimensional phenomenon for seniors. "Aging in place represents a transaction between an aging individual and his or her residential environment that is characterized by changes in both person and environment over time, with the physical location of the person being the only constant" (Lawton 1990:288). Lawton's definition clearly illustrates the dynamic nature of aging in place for both person and environment. Lawton also explains that three types of changes occur as aging in place happens. First, there are psychological changes in the individual over time. Next, the residential environment itself will change due to physical wear, the natural environment, and the behaviors of other people in the environment. Third, changes occur in the process of aging in place based on alterations the resident may make to his or her housing in order to create a more supportive, private, and stimulating milieu. Change is thus a critical notion to bear in mind when discussing aging in place.

More recently, elders are wanting to age in place in environments other than their long-time homes. Many older adults who move to senior housing settings want to remain in these environments and avoid any subsequent moves. Residents hope that services and the physical environment can be altered to meet their changing health needs.

Housing providers have responded to elderly persons' desires to remain in senior housing in one of two ways. One response has been the "constant approach" and the other has been the "accommodating approach" (Lawton et al. 1980). The constant model tries to preserve the original character of both the tenants and the physical environment, to have both remain constant over the years. Within this model, residents are forced to leave the housing setting as their health begins to decline. The ailing residents will then be replaced by new, healthier residents who fit the original ideal proposed for the setting at its inception. The constant approach does not allow for aging in place as it attempts to keep the tenants and the setting static over time. When someone no longer fits the environment, they are asked to leave.

Conversely, the accommodating approach "accommodates administratively by tolerating an extended period of residence of tenants despite growing impairments and by relaxing admission requirements" (Lawton et al. 1980: 62). The facility may assist residents in staying longer by adding more services but this is not necessarily the case. Accommodating environments can occur passively simply by providers allowing residents to stay. Accommodating environments can also occur actively, with providers integrating new services, that declining residents need in order to remain.

The constant approach clearly inhibits aging in place, as was illustrated in the two low service models of assisted living presented by Hawes (1999). Accommodating environments, while more health-care and resident centered, may not actually promote aging in place, but rather what I refer to as "prolonged residence." Prolonged residence means that a tenant can stay in assisted living until some undetermined point in time when s/he needs assistance with four or five activities of daily living (sometimes fewer) or suffers from an unspecified ailment. At this point in time, the liminal phase of prolonged residence is terminated and the older adult is discharged to a higher level of care. Older adults do not know if their tenure in their present housing environment will be five months or five years. Prolonged residence certainly does not guarantee an older adult can remain in their residential environment until they die. While prolonged residence is preferable to being evicted or discharged to a nursing home as soon as they no longer fit the image of an ideal resident, it still places a strain on residents. The reason for this anxiety surrounding prolonged residence can be understood through a brief discussion of anthropological rites of passage.

In cultures throughout the world, rites of passage occur to mark the transition from one stage of life to another. According to Van Gennup (1960), rites of passage have three components or stages. The first stage is *separation*, where the person is symbolically or literally removed from their former status. The second stage is known as *liminality* or the transitional stage. Here the person is suspended between the old role and the new role. Finally, stage three is that of *reincorporation* into the new status or life role. During rites of passage, initiates must learn about the new position they will acquire, its responsibilities and obligations. The liminal, or transitional, phase is considered in the anthropological literature to be the most precarious of the three because the person has no defined role. Turner (1982) further developed the idea of liminality, applying it to any situation in which people are defined as belonging to neither one category nor another. Turner also stresses the idea of *communitas,* or the bonding that the initiates usually experience when they undergo a rite of passage together. Shield (1988) applied these concepts to elderly residents in nursing homes and argued that elderly residents undergo an incomplete rite of passage when they leave their homes and enter the nursing home. The older adults leave behind their role of community-dwelling adult but have no new role to engage in their new setting. Instead, residents remain in this liminal stage, feeling as though they are in a limbo of sorts where they do not really belong. Shield also says that residents do not experience communitas; they do not bond together, even though they are all experiencing the same liminal state. The liminality causes isolation and separation rather than community building.

I argue (Frank 1994; 1999; forthcoming) that residents experience the same incomplete rite of passage in assisted living environments. Further, they endure a heightened sense of liminality because they do not know how long they can stay in assisted living because the facility operates according to one of the varying definitions and models explained previously. Prolonged residence does not allow residents to feel "at home" in their residential environment because their separation from their old status and roles will continue for an unspecified period of time, possibly months or years. The point is that because residents cannot fully age in place (meaning remain where they are until they die), they remain in a suspended state and are very uneasy with this situation. Hence, it is critical to understand that prolonged residence is *not* full aging in place. And while it may be preferable to living in a more restrictive environment, it does not help residents psychologically or socially, as will be explained in greater detail later in this article.

With more and more providers and housing literature using the buzz phrase of *aging in place*, it becomes difficult to know exactly what they mean. In many instances, the marketing literature and trade journals speak of "aging in place" in assisted living but never explain what they mean by this phrase. It is assumed that the reader would know how the phrase is being interpreted. In reality, most marketing literature uses aging in place to mean prolonged residence.

Calkins (1995) explains that definitions of aging in place can be viewed on a continuum of sorts. First, there is the strict official dictionary definition of aging in place that Hawes offered earlier: remaining in one's own long-time residence until death. The next point on this continuum of aging in place definitions would be what is called "a single move." "In this situation, the elderly do not have to move *again* once they have left home and moved to the supportive residential setting" (Calkins 1995:569). The next step on the aging in place ladder would be a scenario of residents remaining within the same building, regardless of health needs. Using Wood Glen Home as an example, an assisted living resident may have to leave the assisted living floor because of increased impairment, but she could continue to live in the building at a higher level of care.

Finally, aging in place has been translated, in its broadest sense, to mean remaining on the same residential campus (such as the case with a Continuing Care Retirement Community). Here, providers refer to their residents as "aging in place" because they do not have to relocate outside of the organization, even though residents may have to move several times within the campus setting (for example, from independent housing to assisted living and then to the nursing home).

A critical question Calkins (1995) asks in relation to this continuum of aging in place is: How do residents interpret aging in place? Calkins points out that most scholars have not addressed this question and, hence, have not addressed the residents' point of view. If older adults fear that they will be forced to leave when they have greater medial needs (at the discretion of the administration of the residence), then their experience is going to be very different than what providers and scholars may think. Before examining residents' thoughts on aging in place, I will first turn to providers' experiences. Since providers set the boundaries for aging in place in an assisted living community, understanding their point of view creates a framework with which to examine residents' experiences.

THE PROVIDERS' STRUGGLE WITH AGING IN PLACE

"Who are suitable candidates for assisted living?" "When is it time for a resident to leave?" These are questions with which every assisted living provider must grapple and both are central to aging in place. None of the ten assisted living sites I visited in the Chicago area had a standard discharge policy written into residents' contracts or marketing materials. This fact reflects the findings of a study conducted by Kathryn Allen (1999). She found that of the 600+ assisted living communities studied, only 48% have resident contracts that specify discharge criteria. Further, in an examination of marketing materials and contracts from sixty assisted living sites, Allen found that twenty of these sites "contained language that was unclear or potentially misleading, usually concerning the circumstances under which a resident could be required to leave a facility" (Allen 1999:9). Since it is by way of these policies that the tension of aging in place becomes evident, it is valuable to examine several providers' verbal policies in order to highlight the complexity of assisted living as a combination of housing and services.

All ten assisted living settings I visited have some sort of criteria for admission into their assisted living program, yet all of these were vague and sometimes contradictory. This, too, is not uncommon among assisted living communities. "Many assisted living providers have poor admission agreements, which resemble real estate property leases more than they do care agreements" (Gordon 1997:39).

Interviews with Chicago area assisted living providers reveal that at one moment administrators are definite about minimum physical and cognitive requirements necessary for entrance into assisted living, then may qualify their answers. An administrator at one Chicago site claims:

> We have certain criteria for assisted living. People must be alert and oriented—but occasional forgetfulness is understood. They must be able to get dressed themselves, for the most part—although we might help them to do a button or a shoe lace or something. They must be continent of bowel and bladder—for the most part . . . they have to be ambulatory, without a wheelchair for the most part.

The above statement illustrates just how paradoxical entrance criteria can be. Some of this vagueness is certainly due to the varying definitions of assisted living. As reflected in Hawes' four types of assisted living, variations between assisted-living types are most often found when deciding how much ADL assistance should be permitted. Some definitions of assisted living in promotional materials do not include any description of assistance; therefore, providers sometimes assume that little ADL assistance will be necessary to them to still be able to call themselves an assisted living residence. Facilities under this heading would likely qualify as one of the "Low Service" models discussed earlier.

Concurrently, providers at Kramer and Wood Glen note the increasing frailty of their incoming population as well as the general decline in their residents over time. According to the social work liaison at Kramer:

> The expectation [at our facility] would be that the residents can take their own medications. We do the shopping, the cooking, the cleaning, the laundry so hopefully the resident can have fun . . . [we want] the residents ambulatory and able to maintain their own ADLs. However, with the change in age of the people coming in–they are more frail and we are providing more services.

The change in residents' health status is more pronounced at Kramer, where administrators and staff have noticed a significant increase in frailty among their residents. According to a nurse liaison for Kramer, family members are noticing this shift as well:

> What I see is even at the family meetings you hear "Has your criteria changed? Are you letting more dependent people in?" But, if you put someone in here at 78 or 80, five years down the road they are going to be 85–*everybody* is going to change. You are all going to decline, unless you are a really active person, and if you are a really active person and able to get around without help, you would not be here.

A problem associated with the increase in resident frailty is the question of what population assisted living is supposed to serve. Every provider interviewed for this study admitted that the health status of applicants had diminished significantly over time. Most providers have, therefore, found themselves altering their expectations and admission standards so that residents may still enter assisted living and stay longer (Frank 1994). However, providers do not want to transform assisted living into a nursing home (Morton 1995). This raises the question of a discharge policy. Removing a resident from assisted living is a very delicate issue, and most providers say that they try to handle such situations based on individual circumstances. At Kramer, the decision is made gradually.

> It is always a case by case decision . . . we have so many meetings before we come to that final decision. We really try everything possible here at Kramer. We usually talk to the family about our concerns, maybe the res-

ident needs more help . . . what we base that final decision on is their cognitive ability–if they are no longer oriented to person, place or time, if they are disruptive to the group or if they cannot really meet their needs, and can we provide a safe environment.

Another Chicago area provider emphasizes residents' abilities to perform activities of daily living as central to their facility's discharge criteria. If the ability to perform one's ADLs is diminished (specifically ambulating and toileting), the resident may be asked to leave.

Usually it is a safety issue. Often it will be repeated falls . . . if there is a problem that sends them to the hospital and when they return, they are at a different level [of care]. Persistent incontinence, and often they will try to hide it.

Providers do try to be compassionate and understanding when it comes to asking a resident to leave. Most respondents say that they really want residents to age in place but are afraid of "over medicalizing" the environment, or crossing licensure boundaries if they are not equipped to do so. The activities director at Kramer poignantly illustrates the conflict.

There is no dividing line–there is no black and white. You are dealing with human beings. I will tell you this, I see Kramer bending over backwards to keep people as long as possible and that is admirable. *However*, that plays havoc with the other residents. It plays havoc because it is a constant reminder of what could happen to them and it is a very real feeling. So, on the one hand, we are trying to keep a resident as long as possible and on the other hand we are hurting the healthier resident 'cause they are constantly reminded at the dinner table how this person's health is declining.

The gray area surrounding an exit procedure reflects the conflict surrounding the issue of aging in place. Regardless of how independent the older adult may be at her time of admission, providers have to know that she will almost certainly deteriorate over time. Negotiating policies that are fair for all parties involved is a difficult task and not necessarily easier for sites that are licensed to offer health-care services. For instance, at Lenington, a Chicago area assisted-living site licensed as sheltered care, providers still have to decide how frail is too frail for their assisted living/sheltered care unit. Administrator Penny Morris relates a story of how she knew it was time for one resident to leave.

We have a lady that was getting up at like 4:30 in the morning so that she would be dressed for 7:30 breakfast. She did not want us to know–her family let us know. She did not want us to know that's how much assistance she was really needing because there is a loss that they feel, if they have to leave sheltered care to go into the nursing home.

After interviewing providers and residents at assisted living sites in the Chicago area, it is clear that these two groups have very different interpretations of what it means to age in place. Most providers interviewed translate aging in place to mean prolonged residence, not full aging in place. Full aging in place occurs only for residents who are fortunate enough to die suddenly of a heart attack or pass away in their sleep. The question remains: are providers hindering seniors from aging in place in assisted living?

My findings show that providers are simultaneously allowing and preventing aging in place. Providers want to allow residents to remain in the homelike setting assisted living offers but, because of confusion about what constitutes assisted living, resident pressures, and state regulations, providers cannot or will not always allow residents to fully age in place. In the short-term most providers in this study were willing to reshape the rules so that a resident may remain in assisted living longer than might have been previously considered "appropriate." Nevertheless, this solution does not resolve the problem of prolonged residence for residents of assisted living.

RESIDENTS' REALITIES IN ASSISTED LIVING

Residents are equally concerned with the question of whether or not they should be allowed to remain in assisted living until they die. A conflict exists for residents because they do not want to be cruel to other residents who become increasingly frail or confused, yet they do not want to be forced to live among significantly impaired elderly. Unlike providers, assisted living dwellers have a much more literal interpretation of aging in place. Based on formal interviews and casual conversations, assisted living residents think that aging in place means remaining where they are until they die, *not* "prolonged residence." As a matter of fact, the policy of prolonged residence makes residents noticeably nervous. A troubling question in their minds is *how long can I stay?* Providers cannot reasonably answer this question. How could they? As illustrated above, every case is handled individually. However, residents see the issue in a harsher light. Residents want to know that they can either stay in assisted living until they die or, that when a *designated* ailment occurs, they must leave. How can older adults feel at home if they do not know how long they can stay? If assisted living is, as one provider claims, "a way station," why would anyone living there feel comfortable enough to call it "home"?

In order to fully comprehend the residents' reality and to illustrate the problems associated with the incomplete rite of passage, it will be necessary to examine their thoughts on activities of daily living–*instrumental,* as well as functional. It will become clear that residents possess a different set of priorities for their activities because they live in assisted living 24 hours a day and are constantly exposed to the declining health of those around them.

As demonstrated earlier, many providers believe that several of the assisted living models should function to relieve residents of responsibilities such as cleaning, cooking, and shopping so that residents can better focus on their health and socialization. These responsibilities are known as instrumental activities of daily living and residents at Kramer and Wood Glen possess a much different perspective on their provision by the facility. They really do not want the "cruise ship" model of assisted living because it compromises their sense of autonomy.

For seniors at Wood Glen and Kramer, instrumental activities of daily living are exactly that: *instrumental* to their sense of independence and usefulness. Many residents state that ADL functioning such as bathing, walking, and eating simply mean that they are alive. It does not mean they are living. Instrumental activities of daily living, on the other hand, represent competence and independence.

Kramer resident Zelda Arnold is perfectly capable of attending to all of her ADLs in her daily routine with minimal help. She says:

> In the morning I go from the bed to the shower, then get dressed, get in the kitchen and get my breakfast . . . then I go out for a walk . . . now I am lucky because I can walk.

At 90 years of age Zelda still accomplishes all her activities of daily living by herself. Nonetheless, these do not give her a sense of purpose or fulfillment. Being denied the ability to perform her instrumental activities of daily living is frustrating for Zelda because she feels she has nothing to do at Kramer.

> I don't have an oven here, I can't bake, I can't do anything! I would like to set up a kitchen that I could work in! I would do my own cooking and not have to put up with whatever they [Kramer] served.

Zelda wants to perform some of the instrumental activities of daily living she was accustomed to accomplishing in her own home. Since the kitchens at Kramer have no ovens, Zelda cannot fulfill her need to cook and bake. Zelda also used to enjoy overseeing her household finances. But this too was taken away from her, not by Kramer, but by her family members.

> I did all of my book work and all my detail work, and when I came here my children decided that it would be too much, so they do all the work. . . . I would like to do all my own book work. I noticed that since I am here, I can't add as quickly as I used to because I was accustomed to doing it every day.

Zelda reiterates the need and desire to participate in her instrumental activities of daily living in order to feel useful and fulfilled.

Tillie Von Deurst, a resident at The Wood Glen Home, claims that many of her fellow assisted living residents constantly complain that there is nothing purposeful for them to do. Tillie jokes, "Complaining is the greatest indoor sport here! I think it is because they [residents] get so bored, you know?" While there are plenty of activities for residents to partake in, activities such as arts and crafts do not create a sense of responsibility or autonomy for people at Kramer and Wood Glen.

Kramer resident George Simon is a veteran of group living arrangements. Before coming to Kramer, he lived in a smaller group living setting consisting of only twelve people. George says, "There, everyone was responsible for something like setting the table or washing dishes. I liked that better than Kramer because doing things like that made you feel useful."

Assisted living residents at Wood Glen and Kramer regard tasks such as shopping and cooking as pivotal to their sense of self-worth because they help define their roles as responsible people. When they moved into assisted living, they moved into a limbo where these responsibilities are handled by staff. Being able to drive or cook or clean gives residents a feeling of confidence and responsibility. For providers, these often appear to be mundane tasks. For residents, these tasks go far beyond merely existing or taking care of ADLs. Residents claim that instrumental activities of daily living, such as shopping or baking, give them active roles in their own lives (Frank 1999; Wilkin and Hughes 1987). And, since the vast majority of people residing in assisted living are women, cooking, cleaning, and washing are activities that these older adults probably performed in their former homes. However, even some men such as George Simon welcome the opportunity to perform such household tasks. He says, "At least here at Kramer, you are supposed to do your own laundry, which I think is good."

Providers at Kramer and Wood Glen often underestimate the critical importance IADLs play in residents' self-perceptions. Providers are frequently oblivious to residents' desires to perform these tasks. Instead, providers are often proud to proclaim that residents' responsibilities are "taken care of." Many providers interviewed in the Chicago area essentially say that their facility takes responsibility for residents' IADLs, such as cooking and cleaning, so that residents can "feel free to relax and enjoy themselves." Residents explain that the only thing they "feel free" to do is to sit and be idle. Having nothing purposeful to do increases their liminality. Providers often view IADLs as burdens and chores, while residents view them as a source of confidence. More importantly, providers are often fearful for resident safety and, therefore, have a tendency to prohibit items such as ovens and stoves from being placed in their facilities. Residents frequently perceive this type of over protection as being treated like children and as a barrier to their IADL fulfillment. Residents in assisted living want their dignity (Heumann and Boldy 1993a). Aside from helping to reinforce one's identity and sense of purpose, performing instrumental activities of daily living can also be what makes a place "home" for its inhabitants. In one's own dwelling, the residents do cook, clean, or pay bills as part of their routine. And, if assisted living strives to be homelike, residents should be able to participate in these home-centered activities if they wish.

Based on the analysis of interviews and field notes from Kramer and Wood Glen, there appears to be a formula that has emerged among the residents. I have named it the *"Usefulness Equation."* This formula is used exclusively by residents for other residents. Providers do not seem to be aware that the equation even exists. The recipe is simple: *IADLs equal usefulness.* Older adults residing at Kramer and Wood Glen perceive themselves as useful and competent only in relation to their ability to accomplish tasks such as cleaning, shopping, driving, cooking, or entertaining, all tasks they formerly completed in their homes. The lack of opportunity to carry out such tasks in assisted living leads them to feel useless. Residents' statements above translate to the notion, "If I cannot do something that I see as useful, then I must not be serving a purpose anymore." Moving into assisted living and discerning no useful roles for themselves amplifies their sense of loss of control over their lives. Residents feel suspended in their incomplete rite of passage. This suspension is highlighted by the fact that residents cannot fully age in place in assisted living and do not know when they will be asked to leave.

Thus far the discussion of residents has focused on how residents see themselves: their own needs, abilities, and sense of capability. An equally important dimension of the ADL/IADL analysis is how residents view each other. This perspective is essential for understanding how assisted living residents feel about the topic of aging in place in assisted living.

"THERE ARE RESIDENTS WHO SHOULD NOT BE HERE"

When talking about their fellow assisted living residents, opinions reveal a double standard regarding aging in place. Tenants at the two sites want to be able to age in place. They need to know that they will not be "thrown out" when they become more impaired. For instance, Wood Glen resident Gertrude Farmer worries about being moved from the assisted living floor to one with higher care.

> If you are independent, you can take care of yourself then you should live here [on the assisted living floor]. But, if you can't and have to be waited on then you have to go up to the third floor [skilled care]. I *dread* to think of that time. I hope that time will never come.

Residents also show this same concern for each other. When talking about other residents, seniors show compassion and concern for cohabitants who are in failing health and worry about them being asked to leave. "It could be me" and "There, but for the grace of God, go I" are common sentiments residents offer about those ailing around them. Still, these healthier residents do not want to see others' impairments on a daily basis. They want to maintain the masquerade of good health as long as possible. The contradictions are evident from the following conversations and interviews.

At Kramer and Wood Glen a number of residents say it is painful for them to witness other residents becoming sicker, more frail, and, therefore, more vulnerable. Yvonne Diamond, Kramer resident, speaks for many of her fellow residents when she says:

> Absolutely, it bothers me. As I said before, I've seen more people get sicker, and I feel sorry for these people. And the thought of their having to go to a nursing home–that alone disturbs me.

While their compassion is strong, so is their criticism. Residents *do not* want to see fellow residents ailing, and healthier seniors voice resentment about having to live with sick people. When entering an assisted living residence, their understanding is that assisted living is for independent seniors. This is not surprising for two primary reasons. First, this opinion mirrors that of providers' initial expectations for assisted living and, therefore, is probably what the senior or family member was told prior to admittance. Second, this perspective is not surprising because at least half of the assisted living sites in the U.S. issue marketing materials and resident contracts that are vague or contradictory in nature, many highlighting the activities and social nature of their assisted living communities (Allen 1999).

Residents wind up measuring themselves against one another. This fact is most evident in the domain of physical health. Many residents say that assisted living should be reserved for "able-bodied" older adults. They harshly contend that many residents at their assisted living sites are too frail to be allowed in assisted living at all. They base such comments on the physical condition of their fellow residents.

Sara Vernon is one resident who holds the view that assisted living must not degenerate into a nursing home setting. Sara, paralyzed on her right side from a stroke, is partially dependent on a wheelchair. She can, however, transfer independently and can walk short distances if there is a hand rail present. In terms of daily routine, Sara is almost completely self sufficient. She has very high standards of independence for all assisted living residents at Wood Glen. She vehemently explains her view of the first floor assisted living wing at Wood Glen:

> I think this first floor [assisted living] is a *mockery!* Because, originally, they had said this was going to be independent. When I say independent, I thought they meant independent except for a little assisted help at times.

Like I need to have my bed made, and I need to have help in the shower. But other than that, no. They have a *diapered person* on this floor and now we have someone who is–well, she is ailing all the time.

Such a response leads one to question what Sara means by independence. She claims it means attempting to do as much as possible for one's self. Sara emphasizes the importance of the *attempt* to do things for one's self.

Wouldn't you *want to do it* [do things for yourself]? If you had to depend upon someone to get a towel or toilet paper? I'll go get it! If I don't know where it is, then I go find someone who will go and bring it to me. I can't see being waited on!

Sara maintains a fiercely autonomous view of how assisted living residents should function at Wood Glen. There is little doubt that her passion is influenced by her own physical constraints as a result of her stroke. Sara wants to fight for independence, and she cannot understand why other assisted living residents would not want to do the same. She was told the assisted living floor would consist of pretty independent residents and is disturbed that this ideal is not the reality. Fellow resident Wendy James takes a similar position as Sara. While being interviewed one afternoon, Wendy lowered her voice and leaned in close to say:

They've got some people here that shouldn't be on the assisted living floor. This woman next door to me–she is sick. (pause) It has upset us to a certain extent. I think the assisted living floor should be as independent as possible. Like, I make my bed, I change my linens. I do everything myself except vacuum and clean the bathroom.

When asked if she likes performing these tasks for herself, Wendy replied, "Yes, I want to feel independent. That way I am my own boss, you know?"

Comments such as these reveal another layer of the IADL/ADL discussion. When talking about their own independence, assisted living residents speak almost exclusively about *instrumental* activities of daily living: making the bed, doing the laundry. Residents like Sara and Wendy measure their personal level of independence based on their ability, desire, and attempts to perform instrumental activities of daily living. When discussing other residents, however, the measuring stick quickly shifts to ADLs. Can the other resident use the bathroom on their own? Can they feed, clothe, or bathe themselves? The inability to perform one's activities of daily living is a sign to other assisted living residents that the individual is not independent and not a suitable candidate for assisted living. The exception to this rule is if a resident (such as Sara) is unable to perform some ADLs, but continues to perform his/her instrumental activities of daily living (such as making phone calls and managing her finances).Then such a person is judged by other residents as at least worthy of residing in assisted living.

Although seemingly cruel, residents at Kramer and Wood Glen should not be viewed as totally uncaring. On the contrary, they care a great deal about their fellow residents and voice genuine compassion about the failing health of those around them. Kramer resident George Simon declares, "It kind of breaks my heart when I see people here with walkers and canes. But, we all have some sort of health problem, that's why we're here." Compassion is evident among residents because they know they have health problems and may also be asked to leave one day. Yvonne Diamond says:

> All you see are people who are deteriorated, and it's hard to see because it is a reflection of yourself too. And, while you know it is going to happen, you don't want it getting thrown at you all the time.

Comments like this are revealing because while residents complain about the disability of others they live with, they also realize that this is why *they* are in assisted living.

Cognitive impairment in particular is one health issue about which residents feel very conflicted and fearful. Cognitively intact residents show much concern for residents who are cognitively impaired, yet are hesitant to live with them in assisted living. Yvonne Diamond relays the following story about a cognitively impaired resident at Kramer. Her concern is clear:

> There is this woman here, this woman who can't see, who can't get around, who can't–she's got Alzheimer's. I pray every day that she does not get hurt on the stairs. Yesterday she got mixed up on the elevator. Now it's time for her to leave, and they [the staff] know this. I'm sure that they are working on something for her. They want to do the best for her, which is good. But see, this woman, well she's senile and [virtually] blind, she goes in and out of it. It is going to kill her when they tell her she has to leave.

Resident Katie Jacobs has a similar story but hers is even more painful because she had forged a friendship with the resident before the woman's dementia progressed. As the resident declined, Katie helped the ailing woman but sensed her friendship role transform into a caretaking role.

> There was one woman, when I came in here–I fell in love with that woman. When I came in here, I liked her so much. I liked her way of looking at things, of living life. And now, she can't remember anything. I took her a couple of times to my room and I changed her blouse because it was on backwards. I liked her so much I would do for her whatever I could. But, how much can I do? So, that is the way it is.

Katie says she no longer socializes with this particular resident.

Despite their own desire to remain in assisted living as long as possible, it is very revealing to find that residents' opinions appear to be more in line with prolonged residence than with the aging in place model. Although residents themselves want to be able to stay in assisted living until they die, they continuously express their preference to live with healthier people now. Residents at Kramer and Wood Glen do not want to watch fellow residents deteriorate. They are clinging to the notion that out of sight *is* out of mind. In effect, they do not have to face sickness and death if it is not there.

At first, residents' contradictory attitudes on the subject of aging in place may seem puzzling. Would residents truly undermine their own potential for long-term residential security by supporting a policy that asks residents to leave, rather than have to be constantly confronted with issues of declining health and death presented by ailing residents? Maybe. The essential choice residents are making is to prioritize their present desire to live among "healthier" residents above their future security of staying in assisted living until they die. Residents choose to hold on to the ideal that they may not decline to the point of eviction rather than face the reality of sicker residents living with them. They are not trying to be cruel when they say "there are people who should not be here." Rather, these people remind them of their own impending vulnerabilities, and they are scared for themselves.

Providers at Kramer and Wood Glen also mention hearing similar comments from residents. They, too, can see residents' conflicts about living with more impaired seniors. Nancy Simpson, social work liaison for Kramer told me:

> I will hear from other residents "This is becoming like a nursing home," "I can't believe this is going on." It's not so much the medical piece on site as much as watching another person deteriorate or seeing companions [for health care services] there [at Kramer]. Sometimes they are very relieved to see the companion [for health care] and know that it can happen to them but they can age in place as well.

The question is, can residents really age in place? Nancy's comments, while potentially reassuring for the present moment, are really more descriptive of prolonged residence. Nancy's statements can really only guarantee them prolonged residence, not aging in place.

Residents know that it is likely that they cannot stay in assisted living until they die; therefore, they don't want to be reminded of their own eventual departure by seeing ailing residents. Their solution: remove frail residents now so they do not have to think about it. Maybe if some of the residents above such as Virginia, Wendy, and Yvonne knew that they were guaranteed a homelike, pleasant, and supportive place to live until they die, they would not be as sure about removing sicker residents. Since all they are guaranteed is prolonged residence, why should they have to witness any impairment in others?

The inner conflict residents face regarding the sickness and decline of those around them speaks to a larger issue: whether or not residents should be allowed to fully age in place in assisted living, meaning to remain in assisted living until they die, regardless of their impairment. Aging in place is the subject of much discussion and debate among many scholars (Sherwood et al. 1990; Tilson and Fahey 1990; Callahan 1993).The aging in place controversy underlies all the questions that both providers and residents grapple with in assisted living. Based on the research at Kramer and Wood Glen, I believe that residents' liminality is enhanced by policies that promote prolonged residence. Therefore, my discussion concludes with an analysis of liminality and prolonged residence as they impact the lives of those in assisted living.

CONCLUSION:
LIMINALITY, PROLONGED RESIDENCE,
AND AGING IN PLACE IN ASSISTED LIVING

Providers interpret aging in place as prolonged residence and add to seniors' sense of liminality and insecurity in assisted living. Since residents do not know what the rules are regarding exit criteria and procedures, they are likely to be more apprehensive about their own failing health. Residents sense this limbo in all aspects of their lives, even in the personal domain, and it increases their isolation. Assisted living resident Gail Young claims, "Nothing here is permanent. So, when you like someone at Kramer, even then you don't get too close because you know that it won't be a long-term thing." This reality does not help residents to feel at home in assisted living. The situation leaves providers with an unsettled feeling, as well. They are struggling just as much with the aging in place issue. According to one assisted living provider in Chicago:

> Most definitely, everybody who is doing elderly housing is dealing with that aging in place issue. And now that we are getting older, more frail clients, we have to be in a position to deal with that.

The question is, how?

Presently, prolonged residence is occurring by default in many assisted living environments. This is because either the provider allows older adults to remain in assisted living by stretching their model of assisted living or because there are no regulations in place yet to force someone to leave at a designated point in time. A major hindrance to the possibility of fully aging in place in assisted living is the perspective of some providers. As shown in comments by several Chicago assisted living providers, too many still view assisted living as a temporary stop along a set continuum of care. Karen Abrams, an administrator at Wood Glen, claims:

The people we have attracted to assisted living pretty much conform to what I expected which would be relatively frail, compromised elderly who might have a good year or two in assisted living but would likely need more supervised care shortly.

Karen Abrams and other providers with this mindset will never get beyond prolonged residence in their assisted living communities. Unfortunately, residents may pick up this unspoken attitude from administrators, thereby increasing their sense of liminality and decreasing their ability to call assisted living "home." Assisted living resident Fannie Isaacs draws a clear connection between the limbo of her life at Kramer and her incapacity to feel at home there. "How can it [Kramer] be home? It is a station before you go there [she points upward]. And, in between you are here."

A strong component of residents' discontinuity is a feeling of uselessness and role loss. They feel suspended: they have no clearly defined role in their assisted living community and do not know how long they can remain there. In their own homes, residents knew better what roles to assume and how they fit in. At Kramer and Wood Glen residents frequently seem lost. Kramer resident Zelda Arnold makes this point very clear in one of our interviews.

> JF: Do you feel like you belong here? [at Kramer]
>
> ZA: Well, I don't know where I belong (laughs). I've got to live somewhere.
>
> JF: Do you feel more like you belong here than at the last senior housing complex you lived?
>
> ZA: (laughs) I don't really know where I belong. When you get to be my age, you don't know where you belong.

Liminality breeds feelings of isolation for a number of residents, and the majority of assisted living models that exist in the United States only enhance these feelings. Assisted living residents do not feel at home in assisted living. The incomplete rite of passage residents undergo when entering assisted living leaves them feeling roleless, frustrated, and bored. Resident Katie Jacobs says:

> I am bored a lot here [at Kramer]. When I am bored I go into my room and watch TV. Sometimes I go into my room when I am bored and I cry, I don't know why, but I cry.

Kramer and Wood Glen residents are very conflicted. They definitely *do not want to see their fellow residents ailing* because they are empathetic and they realize that they, too, will become more frail and then could be asked to leave. Nevertheless, they cling to their liminality by saying: "There are people who should not be here." This is especially true because they realize that they will likely die in a nursing home, the most dreaded place of all (Gubrium 1975; Goffman 1961; Savishinsky 1990). Right now, the only thing prolonged residence offers older adults is prolonged anxiety. Residents do not want this. Seniors in assisted living want to know how long they can stay. They want to know that they *can* stay. Right now, in most assisted living communities, they cannot stay. Therefore, residents struggle to determine what combination of IADL and ADL deficiencies will create the formula for their eviction. The formula differs from one facility to the next, since different facilities follow different models of assisted living. Residents are left to constantly compare their abilities to those of their fellow residents on a daily basis. Identifying those who are "worse off" than they gives healthier residents a temporary sense of security. They think, "after all, if resident 'X' has more ADL dependencies than I do, then resident 'X' will be asked to leave before me." The way to diminish resident liminality and halt the comparisons would be to allow seniors to fully age in place: to stay until they die. However, it must be acknowledged that if residents can remain until they die, they will not be spared the reality of witnessing their cohabitants' decline and death. What they *will* avoid is a sense of insecurity about their own status and having to face yet another move.

According to Victor Regnier, " 'assisted living' is a phrase which means a care philosophy to some people, a building type to others, and to others it defines a regulatory category" (Regnier 1996:1). In order for assisted living residents to have the opportunity to fully age in place, I argue that all three ingredients mentioned by Regnier need to be present in assisted living. Providers must integrate a philosophy of care into assisted living if they want to provide the highest quality of life for residents and honor their dignity. As a building type, assisted living must be residential in character if we want residents to truly feel "at home" rather than institutionalized. Assisted living must also be understood in relation to regulations and standards. Services that can be provided are framed by the regulatory category in which assisted living exists for each state. Residents need to know which health services can and will be provided once they move into assisted living. Developers of assisted living must understand and incorporate all three of these components if there is any possibility of residents completely aging in place.

It is important to point out that an evolution has been occurring over the past decade regarding the level of frailty among assisted living residents. Over all, Kramer and Wood Glen have not remained completely static or rigid in their policies. They are allowing residents to stay longer and utilize more support services. Social work liaison has noted the change at Kramer, a facility that provides no health care services.

I think what is wonderful is when I first started working at Kramer, things were pretty set in that a person had to be independent physically and intact cognitively–alert and oriented. And Kramer only provided the program–which is meals and housekeeping–and that's it. And what I have seen over the years is much more flexibility. Allowing a person to age in place, allowing bathing assistance, allowing a companion to come for maybe three or four hours to help a person.

Kramer still does not supply any health care services, but it allows residents to hire personal care workers to come in and help them. The changes that have been made, while positive, are leading to prolonged residence rather than aging in place. Unfortunately, the situation is problematic for residents because it forces them to deal with ailing residents around them while they are simultaneously unaware of the actual standards for remaining in assisted living.

Perhaps the most positive point to be made about prolonged residence is the fact that it is happening at all. Prolonged residence represents a progression for many assisted living sites across the country. Providers are letting residents stay longer than they did seven or eight years ago. This movement represents an encouraging shift, but it still leaves residents in limbo. Maybe prolonged residence can be seen as a necessary step in the transformation of assisted living from a majority of Low Service/Low Privacy sites to a majority of High Service/High Privacy sites.

Finally, although providers and residents are both conflicted about the aging in place model, there is one important point to bear in mind about the nature of our current elderly housing industry. In the United States the continuum of care penalizes our elderly population for aging. Historically, the more frail and sick an older adult becomes, the *less* homelike her environment becomes. "Industrial society devalues non-productive people, thus when human beings are no longer productive, they become expendable" (Heumann and Boldy 1993a:27). We seem to be sending elderly people in this country a message: *when your health declines you will be moved through a continuum of care into more and more institutional environments, until you end up in a nursing home.* Presently, while a senior may *reside* in the homelike environment of assisted living, s/he is not unconditionally allowed *to stay* in this homelike environment of assisted living until death. Our home is a place which symbolizes security and comfort for us (Lawrence 1987; Rybczynski 1986). How can assisted living be seen as home if providers are evicting residents? Seldom are people expelled from their own homes, yet they can be removed easily from assisted living. Perhaps many providers are interpreting "homelike" merely to mean *the design and decor*, not the philosophy of care.

Thus far, prolonged residence appears to be a shaky compromise for aging in place in assisted living. And, as this article illustrates, it has not worked. Instead, this temporary solution to the growing tension between these two models is having negative repercussions for providers and residents. Providers, researchers, and assisted living advocates must remember that the process of leaving their homes and moving to assisted living is difficult for older adults. "Most older persons are not planning a move, when they do move, they are being pushed out of their previous homes rather than pulled to the retirement housing" (Merrill and Hunt 1990:73). In addition, once pushed out of their old housing into assisted living, residents become suspended in limbo where they give up their old roles without the feeling of acquiring new ones. And, most critically, they give up the certainty of their old environment in exchange for a sense of alienation, few social bonds, and uncertain tenure in their new environment.

NOTES

1. All names of persons and places are pseudonyms.
2. The survey administered to residents was called the Sheltered Care Environmental Scale and was developed by Moos and Lemke (1984; 1988).

REFERENCES

Allen, Kathryn G. 1999. *Assisted Living Quality of Care and Consumer Protection Issues.* Testimony Before the Special Committee on Aging, U.S. Senate, GAO/T-HEHS 99-111, April 26, 1999.

ALFA 1994. *Fact Sheet.* Assisted Living Federation of America. Fairfax, Virginia.

_____1999. *Assisted Living Regulations: A State by State Profile.* Fairfax, Virginia.

Calkins, Margaret. 1995. From Aging in Place to Aging in Institutions: Exploring Advances in Environments for Aging, *The Gerontologist* vol. 35 (4).

Callahan, James J., Jr. 1993. Introduction: Aging in place. In *Aging in Place.* James J. Callahan, editor. Amityville, NY: Generations in Aging Series. Baywood Publishing Company, Inc.

Frank, Jacquelyn B. (forthcoming). *Aging in Place in Assisted Living.* Wesptort: Bergen & Garvey.

_____1999. "I live here but it's not my home": Residents' experiences in assisted living. In *Aging, Autonomy, and Architecture: Advances in Assisted Living.* Benyamin Schwarz and Ruth Brent, editors. Baltimore: Johns Hopkins University Press.

_____1994. Nobody's home: The paradox of aging in place in assisted living. Ph.D. Dissertation, Northwestern University.

Goffman, Erving. 1961. *Asylums.* Garden City, NY: Doubleday.

Golant, Stephen M. 1990. Changing an older person's shelter and care setting: A model to explain personal and environmental outcomes. In *Environment and Aging Theory: A Focus on Housing.* Rick Scheidt and Paul Windley, editors. Westport: Greenwood Press.

_____1992. *Housing America's Elderly: Many Possibilities/Few Choices.* Newbury Park: Sage Publications.

Gordoln, Paul. 1997. When a Handshake Just Won't Do. *Provider,* April.

Gubrium, Jaber. 1975. *Living and Dying at Murray Manor.* New York: St. Martin's Press.

Harris, Diana. 1988. *Dictionary of Gerontology.* Wesport, CT: Greenwood Press.

Hawes, Catherine. 1999. *Shopping for Assisted Living: What Consumers Need to Make the Best Buy.* Testimony before the Special Committee on Aging, U.S. Senate, GAO/T-HEHS 99-111, April 26, 1999.

Heumann, Leonard and Duncan Boldy. 1993a. Aging in place: The growing need for new solutions. In *Aging in Place with Dignity: International Solutions Relating to the Low-Income and Frail Elderly.* Leonard Heumann and Duncan Boldy, editors. Westport: Praeger Publishers.

_____1993b. The basic benefits and limitations of an aging in place policy. In *Aging in Place with Dignity: International Solutions Relating to the Low-Income and Frail Elderly.* Leonard Heumann and Duncan Boldy, editors. Westport: Praeger Publishers.

Kalymun, Mary. 1990. Toward a definition of assisted living. *Journal of Housing for the Elderly,* vol. 7 (1) pp. 97-131.

Kane, Rosalie, and Keren Brown Wilson. 1993. *Assisted Living in the United States: A New Paradigm for Residential Care for Frail Older Persons?* Washington, DC: Public Policy Institute, The American Association of Retired Persons.

Lasky, William. 1999. *Shopping for Assisted Living: What Consumers Need to Make the Best Buy.* Testimony before the Special Committee on Aging, U.S. Senate, GAO/T-HEHS 99-111, April 26, 1999.

Lawrence, Roderick J. 1987. What Makes a House a Home? *Environment and Behavior* 19 (2): 154-168.

Lawton, M. Powell. 1990. Knowledge Resources and Gaps in Housing for the Aged. In *Aging in Place: Supporting the Frail Elderly in Residential Environments.* David Tilson, editor. Glenview, IL: Professional Books on Aging, Scott, Foresman, and Company.

Lawton, M. Powell, Maurice Greenbaum, and Bernard Liebowitz. 1980. The Lifespan of Housing Environments for the Aging. *The Gerontologist* vol. 20 (1).

Merrill, John, and Michael E. Hunt. 1990. Aging in place: A dilemma for retirement housing administrators. *The Journal of Applied Gerontology* 9 (1).

Mitchell, Judith, and Bryan Kemp. 2000. Quality of life in assisted living homes: A Multidimensional analysis. *Journal of Gerontology: Psychological Sciences* 55B (2).

Mollica, Robert, and Kimberly Irvin Snow. 1996. *State Assisted Living Policy: 1996.* Report prepared for the National Academy for State Health Policy, Portland, Maine.

Mollica, Robert, Keren Brown Wilson, Barbara Ryther, and Heather Johnson Lamarche. 1995. *Guide to Assisted Living and State Health Policy.* University of Minnesota: National Long Term Care Resource Center.

Mollica, Robert, Richard Ladd, Susan Deitche, Keren Brown Wilson, and Roberta Ryther. 1992. *Building Assisted Living for the Elderly into Long Term Care Policy: A Guide for States.* A publication of the Center of Vulnerable Populations: National Academy for State Health Policy and the Bigel Institute for Health Policy, Brandeis University.

Morton, Alan. 1995. Camouflaging Care. *Contemporary Long Term Care.* July.

Pastalan, Leon. A. 1990. Designing a humane environment for the frail elderly. In *Aging in Place: Supporting the Frail Elderly in Residential Environments.* David Tilson, editor. Glenview, IL: Professional Books on Aging, Scott, Foresman, and Company.

Pynoos, Jon. 1990. Public policy and aging in place: Identifying the problems and potential solutions. In *Aging in Place: Supporting the Frail Elderly in Residential Environments for the Elderly.* David Tilson, editor. Glenview, IL: Professional Books on Aging, Scott, Foresman, and Company.

Regnier, Victor. 1991. Assisted living: An evolving industry. *Seniors Housing News.* Spring.

_____. 1995. Assisted living models from Northern Europe. *Assisted Living Today.*

_____. 1996. *Critical Issues in Assisted Living.* National Resource and Policy Center on Housing and Long Term Care, USC Andrus Gerontology Center. Los Angeles, California.

Regnier, Victor, Jennifer Hamilton, and Suzie Yatabe. 1991. *Best Practices in Assisted Living: Innovations in Design, Management, and Financing.* Los Angeles: National Eldercare Institute on Housing and Supportive Services, Andrus Gerontology Center, University of Southern California.

Rowles, Graham D. 1993. Evolving images of place in aging and "aging in place." *Generations* 17 (2).

Rybczynski, Witold. 1986. *Home: A Short History of an Idea.* Harrisburg: RR Donnelley and Sons.

Savishinsky, Joel. 1991. *The Ends of Time: Life and Work in a Nursing Home.* New York: Bergin and Garvey.

Shield, Renee Rose. 1988. *Uneasy Endings: Daily Life in an American Nursing Home.* Ithaca: Cornell University Press.

Tilson, David, and Charles Fahey. 1990. Introduction. In *Aging in Place: Supporting the Frail Elderly in Residential Environments for the Elderly.* David Tilson, editor. Glenview, IL: Professional Books on Aging, Scott, Foresman and Company.

Turner, Victor. 1982. *From Ritual to Theatre: The Human Seriousness of Play.* New York: PAJ Publications.

Van Gennup, Arnold. 1960. *The Rites of Passage.* Chicago: The University of Chicago Press.

Wilkin, David, & Beverley Hughes. 1987. Residential Care of Elderly People: The Consumer's Views. *Aging and Society* vol. 7, pp. 175-201.

Wilson, Keren Brown. 1990. Assisted living: The merger of housing and long-term care services. *Long Term Care Advances.* Chapel Hill: Duke University Center for the Study of Aging and Human Development 1 (4).

Wilson. 1996. *Assisted Living: Reconceptualizing Regulation to Meet Consumers' Needs & Preferences.* Washington, DC: The American Association of Retired Persons, Public Policy Institute.

Chapter 2

Residents in Assisted Living Facilities and Visitation Patterns

Dean Thompson
Joseph A. Weber
Kevin Juozapavicius

SUMMARY. Resident visitation patterns within an assisted living facility provide insight into a resident's life satisfaction. This study investigated residents' perceptions of family and friend visitation. Thirty assisted living residents from Oklahoma participated in a comprehensive interview that included demographics, life satisfaction, visitation frequency, and perceptions of visitation patterns. A majority of the respondents (90%) perceived family and friend visitation as "important" to "very important" in their life. Visitation allows residents to reminisce with family members and friends, to fulfill the need to have outside contact, and to be reassured that they have not been forgotten. Results indicate residents do desire continued relationships with family and friends through visitation. Facilities should encourage activities involving outside members of a resident's

Dean Thompson, MS, is Life Enrichment Coordinator, Senior Star Living, Woodland Terrace, 9524 East 71st Street, Tulsa, OK. Joseph A. Weber, PhD, is Director, Gerontology Institute, College of Human Environmental Sciences, Oklahoma State University, Stillwater, OK 74078-6122 (E-mail: jaweber@okstate.edu). Kevin Juozapavicius is Graduate Research Assistant, College of Human Environmental Sciences, Oklahoma State University, Stillwater, OK.

[Haworth co-indexing entry note]: "Chapter 2. Residents in Assisted Living Facilities and Visitation Patterns." Thompson, Dean, Joseph A. Weber, and Kevin Juozapavicius. Co-published simultaneously in *Journal of Housing for the Elderly* (The Haworth Press, Inc.) Vol. 15, No. 1/2, 2001, pp. 31-42; and: *Assisted Living: Sobering Realities* (ed: Benyamin Schwarz) The Haworth Press, Inc., 2001, pp. 31-42. Single or multiple copies of this article are available for a fee from The Haworth Document Delivery Service [1-800-342-9678, 9:00 a.m. - 5:00 p.m. (EST). E-mail address: getinfo@haworthpressinc.com].

support network and be aware of residents less visited, developing programs creating social contact and involvement. *[Article copies available for a fee from The Haworth Document Delivery Service: 1-800-342-9678. E-mail address: <getinfo@haworthpressinc.com> Website: <http://www.HaworthPress. com> © 2001 by The Haworth Press, Inc. All rights reserved.]*

KEYWORDS. Senior housing, life satisfaction, social support

Whether a senior adult lives in an assisted living or a long-term care facility, it is important to examine the amount of social contact the resident receives. For instance, how often are residents visited by family members and friends? What type of visitation patterns prevail? Are the residents impacted by the visitation?

Family members and friends are often seen visiting a resident of a long-term care facility. However, the amount of visitation varies from resident to resident (Regnier, 1995). Some families visit less frequently than others, and some do not visit their relative at all. It is one of the consequences of placement into a long-term care facility.

However, researchers have documented that the majority of elderly persons are not abandoned by family and friends; many maintain social contact through visitation (Hook, Sobal, & Oak, 1982; Shanas, 1979). Thus, the myth of total detachment between a resident and a family member is not always the case. Researchers have claimed that contact is vital for a resident's well-being (Greene & Monahan, 1982). Contact provided by family members and friends can enable a person to cope with stressful events such as a decline in health or the adjustment to a new living environment (Pearlman & Crown, 1992).

Few studies in recent years have investigated the role visitation plays in the life of a resident in a long-term care facility. Previous studies only determined the motivations of a visitor without considering the benefits of visitation for the resident. Consequently, few studies have investigated life satisfaction in relation to family and friend visitation. Furthermore, to date, no study has examined visitation and its benefits among a population of residents living in an assisted living facility.

This study provides an understanding of the value of visitation in assisted living facilities from the perspective of the resident. It is the purpose of this research to reevaluate the role of visitation and its relationship to residents' life satisfaction, thereby obtaining information that will be useful in helping improve the visitor/resident relationship in assisted living facilities. In addition, the size of the social network (the number of family members and friends) of assisted living residents was also examined, and insight is provided regarding residents' perceptions of the amount of visitation and the quality of visits. This research specifically addresses the following questions:

1. Does life satisfaction (LSI-Z Scale) in assisted living residents improve when visitation (number of social contacts) increases?
2. Does the social network size (number of potential family and friends) for a resident increase the amount of visitation they receive?
3. What are the residents' perceptions of the amount of visitation they receive?
4. What are the residents' perceptions of the quality of visitation?

RELEVANT LITERATURE

Visitation

For individuals living in long-term care facilities, family and friends are the primary sources of social support. Maintaining this social support is done through contact with the resident, most likely through visitation. There has been an assumption by researchers that visiting a resident in a long-term care facility is beneficial to the resident (Gubrium, 1976; Hook et al., 1982) by providing the resident social contact with the outside world.

Visitation Frequency. Early studies have determined the frequency of visitation by calculating the number of visits by family members and friends. Most researchers categorized visitation patterns into daily, weekly, monthly, and yearly categories. A nursing home national survey, conducted in the 1970s, revealed that 88% of the residents received visitors occasionally and 12% never received visitors (National Center for Health Statistics, 1979). A study by Kahana, Kahana, and Young (1985) found similar findings with residents receiving at least one visitor per week.

Factors Influencing Visitation. Researchers have assumed that the greater the size of the resident's social support system, the more likely it is that the older person will interact with someone in that support network. Having more family and friends available increases the probability of visitation taking place (Minichello, 1989).

Another factor in determining visitation is proximity. Research has been conducted on the influence the distance between a resident and a visitor has on visitation frequency. Long distances require more time and expense for a visitor making contact with a resident (Minichello, 1989). Not only does proximity reveal visitation patterns, it also explains feelings of obligation by family members and friends to an older person (Montgomery & Hirshorn, 1991). The further the distance between a resident and a family member, the lesser the obligation and the smaller the likelihood that visitation would occur.

Social Support

Residents of retirement villages, assisted living facilities, or nursing homes continue to have support networks comprised mainly of close relatives and some friends (Hook et al., 1982). Social supports are either formal or informal (Bogat & Jason, 1983). Formal support structures are described as social clubs, religious organizations, and government sources; whereas, relatives, friends, and neighbors make up the informal support networks (Bogat & Jason, 1983). Social support networks serve three main roles: they respond to emergencies, coordinate services such as having meals brought in, or act as mediators with the resident's facility (Pruchno et al., 1994).

There is evidence that social support enables an older person to cope better with stressful events, such as the decline in one's health or the loss of a spouse (Pearlman & Crown, 1992). Researchers have found that the individuals who cope best in crisis situations have an accessible informal social support system (Bogat & Jason, 1983).

Life Satisfaction

There have been numerous studies determining conditions that reduce or increase life satisfaction and well-being of older people (Atchley, 1997; Sherman & Wood, 1989). Lower feelings of well-being were associated with the following: poor health, low level of activity, difficulty performing activities of daily living, dissatisfaction with the amount of interaction with friends, dissatisfaction with physical environment, and reduced cognitive capability (Atchley, 1997). Similar results were found in another study which reported that life satisfaction was most influenced by a senior's health (Sherman & Wood, 1989). Other factors reducing life satisfaction were feelings of social isolation and being dependent on others for transportation (Larson, 1978; Sherman & Wood, 1989).

METHODOLOGY

This study was designed to explore current resident and visitor relationships in assisted living facilities. The major purpose of this study evaluates how assisted living residents' visitation patterns relate to the residents' life satisfaction. This study investigates the role of visitation to understand the effects on a resident's life satisfaction and to acquire useful information regarding the visitation from the perspective of the residents.

Participants and Characteristics

The participants in this study were residents of assisted living facilities from five separate locations in central and northeast Oklahoma. The participants constituted a convenience sample and were recruited to participate either by the researcher or the facility's administrators. There were no age requirements or restrictions placed on participating assisted-living residents. Participants ranged in age from 64-97, with a mean age of 83.5 years. There were no gender restrictions; 27 residents (90%) were female and three residents (10%) were male. Twenty-six of the residents (87%) were either widows or widowers, three residents (10%) were married, and one resident had never been married.

Instrumentation

An instrument consisting of an interview and questionnaire was designed to explore the influence of visitation patterns on the life satisfaction of assisted-living residents. The researcher interviewed participants currently residing in the five targeted assisted-living facilities. The semi-structured interviews were broken into three separate sections. During these segments, each resident was asked to discuss his/her basic background, social network size, level of life satisfaction, amount and frequency of visitation, and quality of visits.

Background Information. The first section of the semi-structured interview included 15 questions. Participants were asked a series of demographic background information questions to obtain a profile of the residents.

Life Satisfaction Index Z (LSIZ). In the second section, life satisfaction was measured using the Life Satisfaction Index Z (Wood, Wylie, & Shaefor, 1969). LSIZ is a self-report instrument designed to measure morale. However, in this study the LSIZ was read by the researcher orally to the participants. The LSIZ is composed of 13 statements, asking if the participant agrees, disagrees, or is uncertain about the various statements. The maximum score on the index is 26. An individual scoring high on this index would be regarded as having pleasure from activities, having a meaningful life, feeling major goals have been accomplished, having a positive concept, and having a happy and optimistic mood (Neugarten et al., 1961).

Quantity and Quality of Visitation (QQVS). The final section of the semi-structured interview employed the Quantity and Quality of Visitation survey (QQVS). The survey was designed by the researcher to assess the frequency of contact a resident receives and the participants' perceptions regarding the quality of visitation.

RESULTS

Descriptive Characteristics

The descriptive characteristics of the assisted living resident are presented in Table 1. A profile of the residents indicates that most were highly educated professionals who had lived in their own homes prior to placement.

TABLE 1. Profile of Assisted Living Residents

Categories	N	Percentage
Gender:		
Female	27	90%
Male	3	10%
Age:		
60-69	1	3%
70-79	8	27%
80-89	13	43%
90-99	8	27%
Marital Status:		
Widow/Widower/Single	27	90%
Married	3	10%
Highest Education Level:		
Elementary/High School	6	20%
Some College	16	53%
College	5	17%
Post Graduate	3	10%
Career:		
Homemaker	7	23%
Clerical/Service	5	17%
Professional/Managerial	17	57%
Missionary	1	3%
Number of Months in Facility		
1-6 months	11	37%
7-12 months	5	17%
13-24 months	4	13%
25-48 months	4	13%
49-96 months	6	20%
Residence Prior to Current Placement		
Own Home	18	60%
Retirement Community	4	13%
Adult Child's Home	4	13%
Assisted Living/Nursing Home	4	13%

Relationship Between Life Satisfaction and Amount of Visitation

Resident life satisfaction was measured with the life satisfaction index Z (LSIZ). The theoretical range goes from 0 to 26. The participants' life satisfaction scores in this study ranged from a low of 7 to a high of 25, with a mean of 18. The amount of visitation was determined by the average visits per month for each resident. This amount ranged from 1.8 to 43.6 visits per month, with a mean of 14.3 visits per month.

Relationship Between Social Network Size and Amount of Visitation

Social network size was determined by residents' reports of their total family members and friends. The participants' social network size ranged from 3 to 36 members with a mean of 17.9. The amount of visitation was determined by the average number of visits per month for each resident.

RESPONSES TO OPEN-ENDED QUESTIONS

Residents' Perception of Family and Friend Visitation Patterns

Open-ended questions developed by the researcher were used to assess the residents' perceptions of family and friend visitation patterns. The initial question asked residents if they were satisfied with the amount of visitation they receive. Ninety-three percent of the residents stated that they were satisfied with the amount of visitation. Many of the residents responded affirmatively to this question because they did not want to seem selfish or interfere with their families' lives.

One 83-year-old female, who has resided in the same facility for two-and-a-half years, stated, "I would like to have more company, but I can see what they are doing and how busy they are and if they have time they will visit me, but they have other obligations. If I were to call them to come and see me they would be here for me."

Another question asked if residents would like to be visited more by family members. Fifty percent of the residents did not wish for more visits by family members or stated that they were content with the visits they receive from family members. A 76-year-old resident said, "No . . . I do not want to burden them . . . some people here at the facility talk bad about their children who do not do enough for them, but I am glad my family does not feel obligated to come and visit me." Thirty percent of the residents said they did wish their family would visit them more. The majority of these residents wanted more contact because they had not seen their family members for a number of years. This lack of contact was due to the geographical distance between the family member and resident or to the family member's health condition.

One 81-year-old male resident indicated, "It would be nice to see my brother and sister . . . but it isn't practical, they are unable to visit because of their health and age." Seven percent of the residents wished they could visit their family in their home. Another 7% stated they had not even thought about more visitation by family members.

A third question asked residents to describe the visitation frequency of family members and friends prior to placement in the facility. Fifty-three percent of the residents stated their visits by family members have remained the same since they moved into the facility. Twenty percent stated visitation increased, while 27% stated family visits have decreased in frequency. As for friend visitation, 67% of the residents stated the visits have decreased in frequency. Thirty percent stated they have remained the same, while only one resident stated they have increased. Residents explained the decrease in friend contact as a result of the lack of transportation, moving into a facility away from their own home, and the fact that their friends are experiencing health related problems.

The last question in the interview asked how important it was for the residents that their family members and friends visited them at the facility. Ninety percent of the residents stated it was "important" to "very important" that their family members and friends visit. The reasons the residents gave for their responses revealed several similar themes, such as a sense of connection and emotional support. For example, several residents responded:

- "I would be lost without them."
- "My family is my life . . . that is all I have right now is that touch with the outside world."
- "I would have down days without them . . . especially when I am not feeling well."

Other residents discussed themes of reassurance for family members and residents' role continuity. For instance:

- "I want them to know where I live and see that I am well taken care of and content . . . I think it is important for a family to know, relieving feelings of guilt . . . this makes it easier for them."
- "It is important that I am still regarded as a friend, a parent, and a grandparent . . . I have lived my life in such a way that I hope they want to be around me."

Ten percent of the residents did state they felt it was not important for their family and friends to visit them. One 69-year-old female resident reported, "My family does not get any good out of the visits they give." A 71-year-old female resident, who had lived in an assisted living facility for three years, responded by stating, "It is not important at all . . . I talk to them . . . I do not want to interfere and I do not want them to take off work just to visit . . . they call and check on me and I am satisfied."

Residents' Perception of the Quality of Visitation

Open-ended questions were developed to assess the residents' perception of the quality of visits. These questions centered on the length of visitation, activities participated in during visitation, and the enjoyment of family and friend visitation. The length of the visits residents received ranged from 15 minutes to visits lasting 3 to 5 days.

The residents were asked if they wished the visits were longer or shorter. Fifty-seven percent said they were content with the length of the visits they received. Thirty-seven percent stated they wished the visits were longer, although most understood that their family members had their own lives and did not want to interfere.

Residents were also asked to discuss activities participated in during a typical visit. The residents named twenty different activities (see Table 2). Types of activities mentioned during a visit fell into two main categories: those participated in outside the facility and those occurring inside the facility.

The residents were asked if they enjoyed the visits by their family members. A majority (93%) of the residents enjoyed the visits and discussed reasons why. Comments by residents included:

- "I certainly enjoy the company."
- "I like being around them."
- "Seeing them is nice."
- "I think it is wonderful when your children become adults and can carry on adult conversations . . . there is more of an exchange of ideas."
- "The reason is we start to talk about memories together . . . we talk about when we were younger, times with their father and the funny things we did."
- "I don't know what I would do without them . . . on a day they cannot come something seems really wrong . . . they make life comfortable for me."

The residents were also asked if they enjoyed their visits by their friends. Seventy percent of the residents said they did enjoy their visits, while the remaining 30% claimed they did not have any friends that have visited or had no friends able to visit them. Many residents enjoyed the visits they received from friends because of the things they had in common, revealing a sense of connection, mutual support, and companionship.

One 76-year-old female resident stated, "I enjoy the general conversations . . . it always seems to be a positive input . . . keeping up with physical conditions of others . . . we try to help each other." Similar statements by several residents included, "catching up on the local gossip" or discussing "old times" with their visiting friends.

A common theme with many residents was the decline in the number of friends reported. Many residents stated that they had outlived their friends. However, some residents have developed relationships with younger friends. These residents stated they met most of their younger friends through church activities. An 83-year-old female resident with younger friends reported, "I ap-

TABLE 2. Activities Named by Residents During Visits

Activities	Frequency
Activities Inside the Facility	
Sitting and visiting/Playing games	28
Reminiscing/Looking at old photo albums	6
Inquiring about children's family	5
Visiting with grandchildren, great-grandchildren	3
Visiting other residents	1
Talking about current events/Watching TV	2
Family bringing items needed by resident	6
Family taking care of resident's business	6
Doing laundry with family member	1
Praying with minister	1
Activities Outside the Facility	
Eating at a restaurant	13
Shopping	9
Driving and sightseeing	7
Going to church	2
Going to civic center or meetings	2
Going to movie or opera	1

preciate these young people, because not many do, but there are some and I am glad they are in my life."

DISCUSSION

Few studies have explored the resident/visitor relationship from the perspective of the resident. This study is unique in the evaluation of visitation and the relationship to residents' life satisfaction. Findings help provide insight into the resident/visitor relationship and identify the impact and role of visitation in a resident's life.

It was encouraging to find that a majority of the residents were basically satisfied and content with the amount of visitation they receive from family members and friends. Throughout this research, many residents emphasized that they did not want their family members to feel obligated to visit them. Residents believed making family members feel obligated to visit would disrupt or add burden to their families' lives.

IMPLICATIONS

It is important for family members and friends to understand they have value in a resident's life. Typically an assisted living resident would most likely be adjusting to a new living environment, described as declining in health and having difficulty performing daily activities of living. All of these have the potential to decrease a resident's life satisfaction. Family and friends can enable a resident to cope better and decrease levels of strain and stress. Friends are especially important because they can provide a unique relationship and complementary support for a resident.

Facilities should encourage activities involving residents' family members and friends. This creative programming by senior facilities would encourage family members and friends to participate in a different type of visitation. Facilities should be aware of those residents less visited, as they may be more prone to suffer from depression. Visitation programs should be established to provide a support network for residents to alleviate feelings of isolation.

Senior housing corporations need to know the impact their service has on a senior adult, as well as family members and friends. Researchers and students in the field of aging need to take an interest in studying the influences on life satisfaction for this specific population. It is also important to assess the involvement of the social network of a resident to determine its impact on a resident's life. Social support can enable a senior adult to adjust to life changes, something residents of assisted living facilities continually face.

REFERENCES

Atchley, R.C. (1997). *Social forces and aging* (8th ed.). Belmont, CA: Wadsworth.

Bogat, G.A., & Jason, L.A. (1983). An evaluation of two visiting programs for elderly community. *International Journal of Aging and Human Development, 17* (4), 267-269.

Greene, V.L., & Monahan, D.J. (1982). The impact of visitation on patient well-being in nursing homes. *The Gerontologist, 22* (4), 418-423.

Gubrium, J.F. (1975). *Living and dying at Murray Manor.* New York: St. Martin's.

Hook, W.F., Sobal, J., & Oak, J.C. (1982). Frequency of visitation in nursing homes: Patterns of contact across the boundaries of total institutions. *The Gerontologist, 22* (4), 424-428.

Kahana, E., Kahana, B., & Young, R. (1985). Social factors in institutional living. In W. Peterson & J. Quadagno (Eds.). *Social Bonds in Later Life.* Beverly Hills: Sage.

Larson, R. (1978). Thirty years of research on the subjective well-being of older Americans. *Journal of Gerontology, 33* (1), 109-125.

Minichello, V. (1989). The regular visitors of nursing homes: Who are they? *The Australian and New Zealand Journal of Sociology, 25* (2), 260-277.

Montgomery, R.J., & Hirshorn, B.A. (1991). Current and future family help with long-term care needs of the elderly. *Research on Aging, 13* (2), 171-204.

National Center for Health Statistics. (1977). *The national nursing home survey: Vital and health statistics series 13.* (DHEW Publication No. 43 PHS 79-1794). Washington, DC: U.S. Government Printing Office.

Neugarten, B.L., Havinghurst, R.J., & Tobin, S.S. (1961). The measurement of life satisfaction. *Journal of Gerontology, 16,* 134-143.

Pearlman, D.N., & Crown, W.H. (1992). Alternative sources of social support and their impacts on institutional risk. *The Gerontologist, 32* (4), 527-535.

Pruchno, R.A., Peters, N.D., Kleban, M.H., & Burant, C.J. (1994). Attachment among adult children and their institutionalized parents. *Journal of Gerontology, 49* (5), S209-S218.

Regnier, V. (1995). *Assisted living for the aged and frail.* New York: Columbia.

Sherman, H.J., & Wood, J.L. (1989). *Sociology: Traditional and radical perspectives* (2nd ed.). New York: Harper & Row.

Wood, V., Wylie, M.L., & Shaefor, B. (1969). Analysis of a short self-report measure of life satisfaction: Correlation with rater judgments. *Journal of Gerontology, 24,* 465-469.

Chapter 3

Residential Care Facilities for the Elderly: Toward Understanding Their Place in Community-Based Long-Term Care

JoAnn Damron-Rodriguez
Nancy Harada
James McGuire

JoAnn Damron-Rodriguez, LCSW, PhD, is Associate Director of Education and Evaluation, Geriatric Research Education Clinical Center, VA West Los Angeles and Adjunct Associate Professor, University of California Los Angeles, School of Public Policy and Social Research. Dr. Damron-Rodriguez's research focus is on the linkage of informal and formal services in long-term care. She is a principal investigator on a grant from the UCLA/RAND Center for the Study of Healthcare Provider Behavior, which is studying the relationship of neighborhood crime to the delivery of home health services. Nancy Harada, PT, PhD, is Health Services Researcher, Geriatric Education Clinical Center, VA West Los Angeles, Associate Director of UCLA/VA/RAND MEDTEP Center for Asians and Pacific Islanders, and Adjunct Associate Professor, UCLA, School of Medicine. She is currently studying self-report physical activity measures. James McGuire, PhD, is Director for Research, Social Work Service at the VA Medical Center West Los Angeles and Adjunct Assistant Professor in the UCLA School of Public Policy and Social Research. He is currently involved in evaluation research of housing alternatives for the homeless as well as placement and length of stay in acute health-care settings.

This study was supported by the University of California at Los Angeles Older Americans Independence Center Grant #5p60 A 610415-02.

[Haworth co-indexing entry note]: "Chapter 3. Residential Care Facilities for the Elderly: Toward Understanding Their Place in Community-Based Long-Term Care." Damron-Rodriguez, JoAnn, Nancy Harada, and James McGuire. Co-published simultaneously in *Journal of Housing for the Elderly* (The Haworth Press, Inc.) Vol. 15, No. 1/2, 2001, pp. 43-56; and: *Assisted Living: Sobering Realities* (ed: Benyamin Schwarz) The Haworth Press, Inc., 2001, pp. 43-56. Single or multiple copies of this article are available for a fee from The Haworth Document Delivery Service [1-800-342-9678, 9:00 a.m. - 5:00 p.m. (EST). E-mail address: getinfo@haworthpressinc.com].

SUMMARY. Residential Care Facilities for the Elderly (RCFEs), known as board and care homes, are licensed in California and many other states for non-medical care in the community. RCFEs are examined here to provide illustrative issues in the definition of types of long-term residential care. The research examines physical functioning, social supports, and course of residential placement for 109 RCFE residents (mean age 84 years). A significant portion of the residents had personal assistance needs not usually provided at the RCFE level (75% assistance with medication, 52% used walking aids, 29% assistance in bathing). Additionally, a third of the residents had restricted social supports and social activity. Residents report declines in functioning and support as reasons for moving to residential care. Length of residence in the facility (range less than a year to 15 years) was not related to physical functioning or social activity. These findings do not support "aging in place," within the facility, as the rationale for increased need for assistance in residential care. Implications include the need to maintain the social model of residential care ample for the majority of residents while assuring the availability of a higher need for assistance of a significant portion of the residential care population. *[Article copies available for a fee from The Haworth Document Delivery Service: 1-800-342-9678. E-mail address: <getinfo@haworthpressinc.com> Website: <http://www.HaworthPress.com> © 2001 by The Haworth Press, Inc. All rights reserved.]*

KEYWORDS. Residential care, board and care, formal services

INTRODUCTION

Community-Based Long-Term Care

Community-based alternatives to institutional care are emphasized in the development of long-term care in the United States (Weissert, Cready, & Pawelak, 1995). Yet, as community care options increase, there is a need for unifying concepts, common definitions and terminology as well as distinctions for types of alternative housing (Eckert & Lyon, 1992). Frequently, community-based care is defined broadly as any aspect of care that takes place outside of hospitals or nursing homes (Greene, Lovely, Miller, & Ondrich, 1995). Long-term care is defined as the services that are needed on a continuing basis to enable people with chronic conditions to maintain their physical, social, and psychological functioning, but do not require constant medical monitoring (Harel & Dunkel, 1995). In the less medically oriented community-based care perspective, residential facilities formerly considered as housing or social services now must be examined as components of community-based long-term care and options for residential care differentiated.

Residential alternatives for community-dwelling older adults fall into three major categories: individual, aggregate, and congregate. The social context, as well as the role of both informal and formal supports for elders who live privately or together in housing units, must be considered in developing a more sophisticated framework for community-based care.

The majority of older adults living in the community reside in *individual residences* with three-quarters of persons over age 65 owning their own homes (Gelfand, 1999). Eighty-seven percent of the older persons want to remain in their own homes (American Association of Retired Persons, 1990). These may be their own homes, either an apartment or a house, or the homes of family members. The role of informal supports in maintaining elders in their own homes has been well documented (Noelker & Bass, 1989).

Home health care is the fastest growing component of health care today providing a complement to family support (Hughes, 1992). Increasingly home health care provides high technology medical care in the home as well as supportive services (Arras, 1995). A variety of social services including homemaker services and home modification can enable elders to age in place (Benjamin, 1992). Home health care can also be provided in aggregate and congregate residences as well as private homes.

Aggregate housing consists of retirement communities that provide individual apartments, townhouses, or duplexes that allow residents to maintain their own household, including a kitchen. Only 6% of the population over the age of 65 live in any form of senior housing (American Association of Retired Persons, 1992). This is expected to increase as greater numbers of people age and more housing alternatives are offered (Gelfand, 1999). Aggregate housing ranges from low income public units to private pay for luxurious residences. The numerous households share certain resources, such as recreation facilities, external building and grounds maintenance, and sometimes options for communal dining. Security and safety are strengths of this option. Social activities are arranged or facilitated. Transportation for shopping and medical appointments may be provided.

In contrast, *congregate residency* provides shared living to a greater degree than aggregate housing; this includes communal dining. Among different types of congregate living, individual resident space and services provided vary greatly. More traditional terms for congregate housing have included: domiciliary care homes, adult foster care homes, sheltered housing, and board and care homes. Either congregate or aggregate housing may be provided through public programs established as early as 1937 through the Housing Act and then increased through Section 8 authorized in the Housing and Development Act of 1974. RCFEs fall into this category, which will be described in more detail.

Defining Residential Care Facilities for the Elderly

The increases in residential care facilities (RCFs) require serious attention to their contribution to the continuum of community-based care. RCFs are the most numerous types of residential care. Data from the 1991 National Health Provider Inventory (Center for Disease Control and Prevention, 1994) report 31,431 facilities defined as board and care homes where 413,040 elderly and disabled persons reside. The vast majority of board and care homes are small with 87% having less than 25 residents. Most board and care homes are under proprietary ownership. The western portion of the United States relies most heavily on board and care homes (Center for Disease Control and Prevention, 1994).

RCFs are licensed in California and in several other states are designated as non-medical community care. RCFs provide a supportive living arrangement for people who can no longer reside comfortably in their own homes, but do not require professional nursing care (Bear, 1990). Specifically, the RCF provides a room, meals, housekeeping, and up to 24 hours a day oversight supervision to unrelated adults for a fee (Eckert & Lyon, 1992).

Residential care populations include the developmentally disabled, chronically mentally ill, severely physically impaired, and a growing number of older adults needing assistance. Excluding board and care homes specifically for the mentally retarded, 29.7% of residents were between the ages of 22 to 64, 47% were 65 to 84 years of age, and 21.2% were 85 years and older (Center for Disease Control and Prevention, 1994). Facilities that target residents over the age of 65 are designated as Residential Care Facilities for the Elderly (RCFE).

Mor, Sherwood, and Gutkin (1986) found that nearly one-fourth of the elderly in RCFs need assistance with three or more of their activities of daily living. Informal support networks may meet some functional assistance needs in the RCF environment (Noelker and Bass, 1989). However, questions have arisen related to the appropriateness of these settings for individuals with significant functional limitations or serious medical problems (Hawes, 1994). Further, little is known about the transitions from home or acute setting to residential care (Temkin-Greener & Meiners, 1995).

This research investigates the case for RCFEs as a component of long-term care and the characteristics that require further examination in the development of community-based residential care facilities. This research will describe the characteristics of functioning, social support and timing of placement as important characteristics in defining the level of long-term care for residential programs. Why do older persons enter the RCFE? What are the functional limitations of RCFE residents? What are the formal and informal forms of assistance to RCFE residents? Does need for assistance increase with length of residence and age?

THEORETICAL PERSPECTIVE

Limitations of the research literature on residential care are that it is predominantly regulation and cost focused; has the facility rather than the resident as the level of analysis; and is not grounded in social science theory (Abernathy & Lentjes, 1990; Dobkin, 1989; Stearns et al., 1990). The ecological perspective, based in systems theory, provides a framework for examining levels of long-term care from the vantage point of the person/environmental fit (Greene & Kropf, 1994). Moos and Lemke (1994) have examined environmental performance as determinants of the degree of fit. The degree of fit relates to the individual's ability to perform activities of daily living as well as to their connection to social networks.

The nature of RCFEs' social environment distinguishes them from institutional long-term care settings. Previous research has pointed to the transitional nature of the RCFE social environment. It is a blend of informal and formal characteristics variously described as semi-institutional (Namazi, Ekert, Rosner, & Lyon, 1992), familial (Skruch, 1993; Sherman & Newman, 1988), marginalized (Eckert & Lyon, 1990), and personalized formal relationships (Ekert, Namazi, & Kahana, 1987; Walfson & Barker, 1990). In contrast to nursing home care, all residential care provides a less medicalized and more cost effective form of support for persons unable to live alone (Wilbur, 1994).

Semi-institutional and familial characteristics of residential care are based in the nonprofessional and long-term relationships of staff and residents. Also relevant to the nature of residential care are its relatively open boundaries in comparison to nursing homes. Residents can, based on functional ability, come and go from the facility. Marginalization denotes both the populations served by RCAs and the facilities' isolation from the mainstream of health and social services. RCFs have served persons with long-term disabilities, who are usually poor and whose long-term care needs are not covered through acute care medical reimbursement. Because there is little linkage based on reimbursement, there is a resulting lack of regulation and quality control. These characteristics present strengths and possible weaknesses of RCFs as a component of long-term care. Preserving the social nature of RCFs while assuring that the level of care and quality of service is guaranteed to residents is the challenge.

METHOD

Two proprietary RCFEs in Los Angeles were selected from a list of licensed facilities. These were mid-size facilities licensed for 100 residents. Data collection included face-to-face interviews with residents and facility managers and a review of facility records. A combined number of 109 residents participated. For those residents who were cognitively impaired (Folstein Mini Mental Status score of less than 23), a family member or conservator provided the information. Descriptive statistics delineate the resident population, including former residence and reason for residential placement. Bivariate analysis (Chi-Square) relates background and health functioning characteristics to social support and assistance.

RESULTS

Resident Background Characteristics

The resident population was composed of the very old with a mean age of 84 years and an age range from 62 to 98 years. Seventy-eight percent of the residents were female, 94% were Caucasian, predominantly Eastern-European Americans. Ninety-two percent were currently unmarried. However, most had been married with only 10% having never married. Education was high for this cohort with 32% reporting some college, 23% high school graduation, 17% some high school, and 20% eighth grade education or less (8% missing data). Approximately 28% received Supplemental Security Income and Medicaid and were, thus, low income. (See Table 1.)

Thirty-four percent of the residents reported having no family. Thirty-seven percent of the residents reported having daughters and sons as their primary family contact. Sisters and/or brothers were the primary family contact for 6% of the residents. Only 1% identified a spouse, and the remaining 22% listed other unspecified family contacts. Ninety-two percent of the residents' primary family contacts lived within the state.

Health and Functioning

The self-reported health of the residents ranged from excellent to poor with 69% reporting good to excellent health and 32% reporting fair to poor health. The following are the reported rates of need for assistance in activities of daily living (ADLs): 29% bathing, 12% dressing, 4% toileting, 3% feeding. Seventy-three percent of the residents were assisted with medication by facility staff. Almost half of the residents used walking aids, either walkers or canes.

Fifty-four percent of the residents were not hospitalized in the previous year, 33% were hospitalized once, and 14% more than once. Seventy percent of the residents saw a physician more than once last year, 29% visited the doctor only once, and 4% had no physician contact last year.

Previous Living Arrangement and Reason for RCFE Move

Seventy-five percent of the RCFE residents moved to the facility from their own home. Ten percent moved to the RCFE from the home of another person, 7% had been living in another residential care facility, 2% moved to the facilities post hospitalization, none of the residents moved to the facility after nursing home placement, and 6% listed a variety of other living arrangements, such as senior apartments, prior to the RCFE move. (See Figure 1.)

Reasons for moving to the RCFE were predominantly declines in functioning and social support. Forty-seven percent stated problems in caring for themselves, 23% reported a decrease in family support, 11% noted the lack of socialization, and 2% recognized problems in managing their finances. Length of residence in the facility ranged from less than 1 year to 15 years with a mean of 3.5 years and a median of 2.6 years. (See Figure 2.)

Social Activity

Social activity participation within the facilities was high; 72% of the residents were involved on a weekly basis. Six percent were only active in facil-

TABLE 1. RCFE Resident Characteristics
(N = 109)

Age (years)		
Mean	84	
Range	62-98	

	%	(n)
Gender		
Female	78	85
Male	22	24
Marital Status		
Married	8	9
Widowed	66	72
Divorced/Separated	13	14
Never Married	10	11
Missing	3	3
Race		
Caucasian	94	102
Other	6	7
Education		
8th Grade or Less	20	22
Some H.S.	17	18
H.S. Grad.	23	25
College	32	35
Missing Data	8	9
Income		
Private Pay	72	78
SSI	28	31

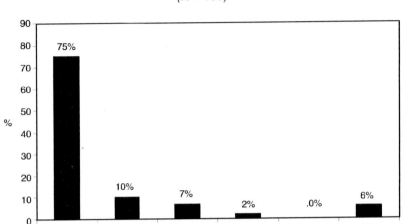

FIGURE 1. Previous Living Arrangement of RCFE Residents
(N = 109)

ity-based activities on a monthly basis, and 22% reported never participating. Fifty-five percent of the residents leave the facility at least weekly, 14% leave the facility at least monthly, but 32% are facility bound.

Forty-three percent of the residents visited with friends weekly or more, while 9% visited friends only monthly. Forty-eight percent reported having no contact with friends. Fifty-one percent visited with family weekly or more, 19% monthly, and 27% had no family contact. Nineteen percent reported receiving help from family in walking, and 27% received informal support in other areas of aid.

In bivariate analysis, age, gender, race, education and SSI were not significantly related to functional needs or assistance. Use of walking aids was significantly related to not leaving the RCFE for social activity (p > .05). Needing assistance in bathing was significantly related to hiring formal help (p > .001). Age was not related to length of residence, and length of residence was not related to need for assistance.

DISCUSSION AND IMPLICATIONS

This research adds to the small body of studies that investigate residential care at the level of the resident. However, it is limited by its small sample size and the non-random selection of facilities. It does point to three areas requiring

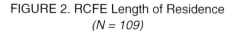

FIGURE 2. RCFE Length of Residence
(N = 109)

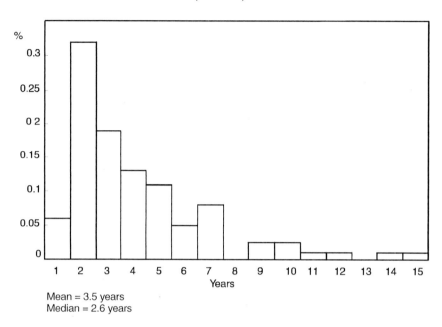

Mean = 3.5 years
Median = 2.6 years

further investigation: (1) the heterogeneity of the residential care population particularly focusing on those who could benefit from increased personal assistance, (2) the mix of informal and formal supports in residential care and (3) the trajectory or course of residential placement.

Resident Assistance Needs

The majority of residents studied do not require long-term care services above those normally provided in residential care: housekeeping, meal preparation, and general supervision. This is supported by their self reported health: 69% of the residents rated their health as good or excellent. This supports the need for the social model of care currently provided by the RCFE or board and care.

However, almost one-third (29%) required assistance with one or more ADLs. The highest ADL need was for bathing assistance. This need in bathing was strongly related to residents hiring formal assistance. Additionally, more than two-thirds (73%) of the residents received assistance with their medications. A third of the residents were hospitalized at least in the last year. The need for assistance found in this research is less than in earlier research that found nearly one-fourth of the residents needing assistance with 3 or more of their activities of daily living (Mor, Sherwood, & Gutkin, 1986). Even for those who required more assistance than normally provided in the RCFE, the majority did not meet criteria for nursing home care. Only three percent of the resident population was possibly at risk of nursing home care based on their need in four ADLs, including feeding.

To maintain the social model of care and not unduly medicalize the environment of the RCFE, the specific needs of the elderly must be personalized. The mix of higher functioning and frailer residents may be a strength of residential care. Moos and Lemke view diversity of residents and staff as a strength of the social climate in residential care (1994). Residents dependent on walking aids were less likely to leave the facility and its architectural modifications such as those seen in the best practices described by Regnier, Hamilton, and Yatabe (1991).

Assisted living has emerged as an alternative for persons requiring significant levels of personal care and yet not needing the 24 hour skilled care in a nursing home (Wilson, 1993; Yee, 1993). There are over 700 assisted-living facilities in the United States (Assisted Living Facilities Association of America, 1995). This relatively new option is defined as "any group residential programs that are not licensed as a nursing home that provides personal care to persons with need for assistance in the activities of daily living (ADLs), and that can respond to unscheduled needs for assistance that might arise" (Kane & Wilson, 1993). At least one-third of the residents in this study could not afford more expensive residential care. Those requiring assistance with bathing were likely to be paying out of pocket for that help. These new assisted-living arrangements are frequently entrepreneurial ventures for older persons who can privately pay for enhanced service, and there is concern for those unable to bear this cost (Reschovsky & Ruchlin, 1993).

Public services may be an effective means of providing assisted living services for low income elderly. This "patch" of Title XX, Department of Public Social Service, in home supportive services would allow for a segment of the RCFE population at risk of nursing home placement to continue to live in a more social environment (Sheehan, 1994). Based on a statewide survey of board and care facilities in Maryland, the increased match of resident to residential facility and community services was a strong recommendation (Dobkin, 1989) from the American Association of Retired Persons (AARP).

Informal and Formal Supports

The research supports that the majority of older adults living in RCFE settings are socially active, but approximately one-third were isolated from contact outside the facility and did not participate in social activities within the facility. In contrast, about one-third have regular contact and assistance from family, and the remaining one-third had more limited social supports.

Litwak (1985) has distinguished the difference between informal and formal assistance. The blurring of these roles in RCFE care is an important area for further exploration in community-based care. Informal care based on affection, social interaction, filial ties, and knowledge of the person over time may fall along a continuum. Caring for a spouse at home may be at the most intense level of informal care, but an RCFE staff member caring for an elder in a small facility for as many as 15 years may also be more of the nature of informal than formal care. Yet as the care needs increase for elders in residential care, the need for formal services based in professional knowledge and skill may be required in either of these settings.

Interviews with family caregivers would be valuable supplements to reports of residents and RCFE managers. Within the context of informal supports, cultural and ethnic factors should be considered in future research. Though ethnicity was not a focus of this research, it should be noted that the majority of the residents were Eastern European immigrants, an element that may relate not only to informal support but also to other elements of the social climate of the facility and personal adjustment to residential care.

Residential Care Trajectory

The older persons in this study moved to the RCFE from their own homes and to a lesser extent from the homes of other persons. It is noteworthy that few were placed in residential care after an acute hospitalization, and no elder reported coming to the RCFE from a nursing home. These are self and RCFE operator reports of previous residence. The role of discharge planners and health care professionals in referring to residential care is not known. Forty-three percent of the residents reported declines in functioning as reasons for moving to the RCFE. At critical junctures in the elderly's care trajectories are residential care options considered as an alternative to returning home or going to a nursing home?

No significant relationship was shown between age and length of residence in the RCFE. Length of residence did not relate to decrease in functioning or need for assistance. Residents reported loss of functioning in their home setting as the major reason for moving to the RCFE. These findings suggest that the "aging in place" phenomenon may be the reason for the move to residential living rather than the reason for additional assistance in the placement. The decline in functioning may occur in the private residence and necessitate the move to residential housing. However, the decline did not necessitate 24 hours a day nursing home care. The trajectory or course of service use is an area of needed study to understand the use of long-term care services over time. Future research should examine the pattern of functional decline before and after residential placement. Programs and practice implications include the need to plan and consider residential placement options at different junctures in late life. RCFEs may provide a first step in a continuum of need or may be all that is required in the way of assistance as shown by the elders who lived for as long as 15 years in the RCFE without requiring additional aids. Physicians and other health professionals who play a role in long-term care planning should be made more aware of residential care resources and their limitations.

CONCLUSION

Residential care provides an important foundation level of support in the continuum of community-based long-term care. For many elderly, it may supply the safety net needed for living in the community with more increased support than the norm of independent living in the home or aggregate senior housing. For a significant portion of older adults, who do not require the medical care provided in a nursing home, but do need more personal assistance than usual RCFE services, more innovative approaches such as those provided in assisted living are desirable. Policies and programs must consider the cost of added assistance since residential care is currently on the margin of health care and not a covered medical benefit. Innovative approaches for public funding must be explored if assisted living is to be available to the low income elderly. Providing additional assistance should be done within the social model of care which integrates informal supports and community access because these are strengths of the RCFE level of long-term care.

REFERENCES

Abernathy, T.J., & Lentjes, D.M. (1990). A three year census of dependent elderly. *Canadian Journal of Public Health,* 81 (1): 22-26.

American Association of Retired Persons (1990). *Understanding Senior Housing for the 1990's.* Washington, DC: Author.

Arras, J.D. (1995). *Bringing the Hospital Home: Ethical and Social Implications of High-Tech Home Care.* Baltimore, Maryland: The John Hopkins Press.

Assisted Living Facilities Association of America (1995). *Assisted Living.* Fairfax, Virginia: Author.

Bear, M. (1990). Social networks: Impact on returning home after entry into residential care homes. *The Gerontologist,* 30 (1), 30-34.

Benjamin, A.E. (1992). An overview of in-home health and supportive services for older persons. In Marcia Gory and Alfred P. Duncker (Eds.) *In-Home Care for Older People: Health and Supportive Services.* Newbury Park: Sage.

Center for Disease Control and Prevention (1994). *Nursing Homes and Board and Care Homes: Data for the 1991 National Provider Inventory.* No. 244. Washington, D.C.: U.S. Department of Health and Human Services.

Dobkin, L. (1989). *The Board and Care System: A Regulatory Jungle.* Washington, DC: American Association of Retired Persons.

Eckert, J.K., Namazi, K.H., & Kahana, E. (1987). Unlicenced board and care homes: An extra-familial living arrangement for the elderly. *Journal of Cross-Cultural Gerontology,* 2, 377-393.

Eckert, J.K., & Lyon, S.M. (1991). Regulation of board and care homes: Research to guide policy. *Journal of Aging & Social Policy, 3* (1-2), 147-162.

Eckert, J.K. & Lyon, S.M. (1992). Board and care homes: From the margins to mainstream in the 1990s (97-114). In Marcia G. Ory & Alfred P. Dunker (Eds.) *In-Home Care for Older Persons.* Newbury Park: Sage.

Gefland, D.E. (1999). *The Aging Network: Program and Services.* New York: Springer Publishing Company.

Greene, R., & Kropf, N. (1994). Ecological assessment and intervention. A presentation at the Annual Meeting of the Gerontological Society Annual Meeting in Atlanta, Georgia.

Greene, V.L., Lovely, M.E., Miller, M.D., Ondrich, J.I. (1995). Reducing nursing home use through community long-term care: An optimization analysis. *Journal of Gerontology: Social Sciences,* 50 (4): S259-S268.

Harel, Z., & Dunkle, R.E. (1995). *Matching People with Services in Long-Term Care.* New York: Springer Publishing.

Hawes, C. (1994). New board-and-care role raises quality-of-care concerns. *Aging Today.* March/April, 17.

Hughes, S.L. (1992). Home care: Where we are and where we need to go (54-75). In Marcia G. Ory & Alfred P. Dunker (Eds.) *In-Home Care for Older Persons.* Newbury Park, CA: Sage Publications.

Kane, R.A. & Wilson, K.B. (1993). Assisted Living in the US: A New Paradigm for Residential Care for Frail Older Persons? Washington, DC: Public Policy Institute, American Association of Retired Persons.

Litwak, E. (1985). *Helping the Elderly.* New York: The Guilford Press.

Moos, R., & Lemke, S. (1994). *Group Residence of Older Adults: Physical Features, Policies and Social Climate.* New York: Oxford University Press.

Mor, V., Sherwood, S., & Gutkin, C. (1986). A national study of residential care homes serving the elderly patients. *Journal of Gerontology,* 40, 164-171.

Namazi, K.H., Eckert, K., Rosner, T.T., & Lyon, S. (1991). The meaning of home for the elderly in pseudo-familial environments. *Adult Residential Care Journal* 5: 81-96.

Noelker, L.S., & Bass, D.M. (1989). Home care for elderly persons: Linkages formal and informal caregivers. *Journal of Gerontology: Social Sciences,* 44 (2): S63-S70.

Regnier, V., Hamilton, J., & Yatabe, S. (1991). *Best Practices in Assisted Living: Innovations in Design, Management and Financing.* Los Angeles: National Eldercare Institute on Housing and Supportive Services, Andrus Gerontology Center, University of Southern California.

Reschovsky, J.D., & Ruchlin, H.S. (1993). Quality of board and care homes serving low-income elderly: Structural and public policy correlates. *The Journal of Applied Gerontology, 12,* 2, 245-254.

Sheehan, N.W. (1994). Bringing together housing and aging services: The experiences of Area Agencies on Aging. A presentation at the Annual Meeting of the Gerontological Society of America, Atlanta, GA.

Sherman, S.R., & Newman, E.S. (1988). *Foster Families for Adults.* New York: Columbia University Press.

Skruch, M.K. (1993). *Family-likeness in the Small Board and Care Home: The Measurement and Prediction of the Interpersonal Environment.* PhD Dissertation, Policy Sciences Department, University of Maryland.

Stearns, L.R., Netting, F.E., Wilson, C.C., & Branch, L.G. (1990). Lessons from implementation of CCRC regulation. *Gerontologist,* 30 (2): 154-61.

Temkin-Greener, H., & Meiners, M.R. (1995). Transition in long-term care. *Gerontologist,* 35 (2), 196-206.

Weissert, W., Cready, C.M., & Pawelak, H. (1988). The past and future of home and community based long-term care. *The Milbank Quarterly,* 66: 309-388.

Wilbur, V. (1994). Enhancing options. *Provider,* 20 (3): 61-62.

Wilson, K.B. (1993). Assisted living: A model of supportive services. *Advances in Long-Term Care.* New York: Springer Publishing Co.

Yee, D.L. (1993). *Final Report: Ensuring Resident-Centered Care in Assisted Living.* Waltham, MA: Report of the Commonwealth Fund (Grant No. 93-78).

Chapter 4

Residential Care Supply and Nursing Home Case Mix

Robert Newcomer
James Swan
Sarita L. Karon

SUMMARY. An evolution is occurring in state policy and industry practices relative to assisted living and expanded use of residential care facilities (RCFs) for persons with physical and cognitive frailty, yet relatively little is known about the interrelationship between this housing supply and nursing home case mix. This article summarizes an analysis of these relationships. The findings raise caution about the optimistic assumptions of the interplay between RCF policy and nursing home use. The proportion of nursing home cases with only physical and cognitive impairment likely to be affected by emerging long term care policy appears to be much less than 25%. *[Article copies available for a fee from The Haworth Document Delivery Service: 1-800-342-9678. E-mail address: <getinfo@ haworthpressinc.com> Website: <http://www.HaworthPress.com> © 2001 by The Haworth Press, Inc. All rights reserved.]*

KEYWORDS. Residential care, assisted living, nursing homes, long-term care

Robert Newcomer is affiliated with University of California, 3333 California Street, Suite 455, San Francisco 94143-0612 (E-mail: rjn@itsa.ucsf.edu.) James Swan is affiliated with Wichita State University. Sarita L. Karon is affiliated with University of Wisconsin, Madison.

Funded by the Commonwealth Fund, grant number 96611.

[Haworth co-indexing entry note]: "Chapter 4. Residential Care Supply and Nursing Home Case Mix." Newcomer, Robert, James Swan, and Sarita L. Karon. Co-published simultaneously in *Journal of Housing for the Elderly* (The Haworth Press, Inc.) Vol. 15, No. 1/2, 2001, pp. 57-66; and: *Assisted Living: Sobering Realities* (ed: Benyamin Schwarz) The Haworth Press, Inc., 2001, pp. 57-66. Single or multiple copies of this article are available for a fee from The Haworth Document Delivery Service [1-800-342-9678, 9:00 a.m. - 5:00 p.m. (EST). E-mail address: getinfo@haworthpressinc.com].

Analyses of a national sample of nursing home populations suggest that between 25% and 35% of the one million plus nursing home residents are there due mainly to limitations in the ability to perform such personal care tasks as bathing, dressing, and ambulation (Spector, Reschovsky, & Cohen, 1996). How to move such individuals into assisted living or other types of supportive housing or how to prevent them from entering nursing homes are compelling challenges to state government. To do this, states have adopted policies to constrain nursing home growth, have stimulated the growth of the assisted living bed supply, have extended access to assisted living by reshaping eligibility criteria, and have provided financial reimbursement for home- and community-based care (e.g., homemakers, personal care aides) that may be needed in such housing (Mollica, 1998). Yet, it remains undetermined how many nursing home residents might actually shift to alternative settings.

This article summarizes the results of a Commonwealth Fund sponsored study that used nursing facility and county-level data to assess the relationship between licensed supportive housing supply and nursing home case mix in five states (Newcomer, Swan, Bigelow et al., 1999). Findings from these models were also used in a simulation analysis illustrating how nursing home case mix might be affected if the conditions in one state are adopted by others.

METHODS

The principal data sources for these analyses were the OnLine Survey, Certification, and Reporting System (OSCAR); and the nursing home Minimum Data Set (MDS). OSCAR data include facility characteristics (e.g., size, ownership, and age) and staffing. The MDS is specific to each resident, measuring functional abilities, medical problems, and emotional states (such as depression and behavior problems). MDS data were pooled to classify a facility's case mix. OSCAR and MDS data were supplemented to include community or market area characteristics. These data were obtained from the Area Resource File, which is a compilation of census and other county level data assembled by the Bureau of Health Professions, Department of Health & Human Services. The data elements pertain to 1995 or reflect governmental estimates for 1995, the period used for the MDS and OSCAR data. Residential care beds (defined to include all elderly supportive housing licensed by the state, regardless of the term used by each particular state to describe its supportive housing) data were obtained directly from state licensing and regulatory agencies in each state. Unlicensed supportive housing facilities were not enumerated in these analyses.

Five states (Kansas, Maine, Mississippi, Ohio, South Dakota), compiling MDS data into statewide data systems in 1995, were used in these analyses, providing a total of 1,555 freestanding nursing homes (the unit of analysis). Complete OSCAR and MDS records were matched for 95.4% of these facilities. Hospital-based nursing facilities were not included in the analysis, nor were facilities serving only the mentally ill. The states, as shown in Figure 1, reflect a spectrum of state policies relative to nursing homes and residential care, and varying market conditions.

Resource Utilization Groups, version III (i.e., RUG-III), were used to consolidate resident characteristics into a standardized case mix classification sys-

FIGURE 1. Summary of State Policies Affecting Nursing Home and Residential Care Eligibility and Financing, 1995

	Kansas	Maine	Mississippi	Ohio	South Dakota
PAS Screening	Required of all nursing facility admissions, prior to and including 1995	Required of all nursing facility admissions only after 10/1/1995	Minimal screening of nursing facility admissions prior to and during 1995	Required of all nursing facility admissions only after 1/1995	Required of all nursing facility admissions since 1988
Nursing facility eligibility criteria	3+ADL + 2+IADL & other skilled care needs	3+ADL + daily skilled nursing or 5x per week therapies	3+ADL or other skilled nursing or therapy need	3+ADL or other skilled care need	24 hour supervision or skilled nursing need
Medicaid funds for residential care	HCBC, 1995	None, 1995	None, 1995	None, 1995	Up to $150/month available in some RCFs
SSP or other state funds for residential care	Up to $155 monthly	$49-$219, 1995	None, 1995	None, 1995	Up to $250 monthly available in some RCFs
Residential care eligibility	Screening only if HCBC	No exclusions, home health care required for those needing skilled nursing	Ambulatory, continent, non violent	Few exclusions; up to 100 days or more of intermittent nursing permitted	Excludes residents who need more than limited hands-on physical assistance or who require on-going nursing

PAS refers to pre-admission screening of those applying for nursing facility placement. ADL refers to activities of daily living; IADL refers to instrumental activities of daily living. SSP refers to state supplemental payments to the federal minimum income subsidy program known as Supplemental Security Income (or SSI). HCBC refers to the home and community-based care program, funded by states under waivers to the Medicaid program.

tem. These classifications are based on assessment data in the nursing home Minimum Data Set (MDS). The major RUG-III hierarchical classifications shown below were used (Fries, Schneider, Foley et al., 1994). Residents were classified by their most resource intensive group. Two sets of case mix classifications were compiled for each facility. One used the MDS records of admissions during the calendar year. The second represented the continuing or average daily case mix in the facility.

- *Rehabilitation (Special).* Residents receiving physical, occupational, or speech therapy with the treatment goal of restoring function define this classification.
- *Extensive Care.* Residents with a RUG-III ADL Index score of at least 7 (on a scale that ranges from 4 to 18 points) and who require one or more of the following: parenteral feeding, suctioning, tracheostomy, or respirator/ventilator care.
- *Special Care.* Residents with a RUG-III ADL Index score of at least 7 and one or more of the following serious conditions: burns, coma, fever (with vomiting, weight loss, pneumonia, or dehydration), multiple sclerosis, stage 3 or 4 pressure ulcers, quadriplegia, septicemia, intravenous medications, radiation treatment, tube feeding.
- *Clinically Complex.* Residents with at least one of the following: aphasia, aspirations, cerebral palsy, dehydration, internal bleeding, hemiplegia, pneumonia, stasis ulcer, terminal illness, urinary tract infection, chemotherapy, dialysis, 4+ physician visits per month, respiratory or oxygen therapy, transfusions, wound care other than pressure ulcer care (including active foot dressings). Patients meeting Extensive or Special Care criteria, but with RUG-III ADL Index scores of 4-6, are also classified as Clinically Complex.
- *Cognitively Impaired.* Residents with a RUG-III ADL Index score of 4-10 and with cognitive deficits in all three of the following: short-term memory, orientation, and decision making. Persons with a combination of both cognitive impairment and behavior problems are classified as cognitively impaired.
- *Behavior Problems.* Residents with a RUG-III ADL Index score of 4-10 and displaying daily problems with inappropriate behavior, physical abuse, verbal abuse, wandering, or hallucinations.
- *Physical Functions.* Residents not meeting the conditions for any of the previous categories, but who have a RUG-III ADL Index score of 11 or more.

Among the more than 1,500 nursing homes used in this analysis, the most common resident classifications were: "Clinically Complex," accounting for a third to a half of all residents; "Physical Problems," accounting for about 20% to 40% of residents; and "Cognitive Impairment," about 10% to 15% of residents. Individuals in these latter two groups reflect those whose needs are predominantly for personal care. The balance of residents includes those with behavioral problems and those receiving rehabilitation or other forms of skilled care. The prevalence rates for those with personal care needs are consistent with the previously cited estimates (Spector et al., 1996) and may suggest an upper bound on the proportion of the current nursing home population potentially served in supportive housing. (See Table 1.)

FINDINGS

Among the assumptions underlying the adoption of less restrictive state RCF policy are that consumers will have more choice in where they live and that the state may experience reduced demand for Medicaid reimbursed nursing home stays. Two case mix outcomes were expected:

- The proportions of *skilled* care patients in nursing facilities (e.g., rehabilitation, extensive, special, clinically complex care) will be higher in those communities where relatively frail custodial patients could (either by policy or financing) receive care in RCFs. This proposition assumes either sufficient demand for skilled care and/or that nursing home occupancy will be lower as fewer of the custodial care patients remain in these facilities.
- The proportions of frail custodial patients in nursing facilities (e.g., cognitive impairment, behavior problems, physical impairment) will be lower in those communities where custodial patients could (either by policy or financing) receive care in RCFs. This proposition also assumes sufficient demand for skilled care to replace custodial cases and/or that nursing home occupancy will be lower as fewer of custodial care patients remain in these facilities.

The findings (reported in-depth in Newcomer, Swan, Bigelow et al., 1999) suggest that facilitative reimbursement for RCF care (within the very modest payments offered by three states) and relatively non-restrictive RCF eligibility criteria, whether occurring together or separately, were not sufficient to substantially affect nursing home demand at admission during the observed period. Demand was expressed by case mix and occupancy rate. This finding holds regardless of the relative supply of nursing home beds in a community or the relative supply of RCF beds. For continuing care (again in the context of non-restrictive RCF eligibility and some financing), nursing facility case mix seems to be affected by RCF competition only in communities having a relatively high proportion of nursing facilities per population. Table 2 shows the descriptive statistics for the variables included in the analysis.

TABLE 1. Case Mix at Time of Nursing Facility Admission and Averaged Over Calendar Year 1995–Freestanding Facilities Only

Average Percentages Across Facilities

Percentage of Residents in RUG-III Classifications	Kansas (n = 366)	Maine (n = 121)	Mississippi (n = 142)	Ohio (n = 754)	South Dakota (n = 94)
Admission Case Mix					
% Rehabilitation	7.19	9.08	3.47	10.73	2.18
	(11.99)	(10.65)	(7.13)	(14.47)	(4.78)
% Extensive	0.76	1.05	2.01	2.29	1.34
	(2.26)	(1.96)	(3.51)	(5.04)	(3.07)
% Special Care	6.04	7.51	11.70	9.40	12.52
	(8.40)	(6.43)	(7.97)	(9.09)	(13.36)
% Clinically Complex Care	33.44	45.09	38.09	48.82	48.08
	(20.19)	(17.58)	(13.67)	(17.79)	(20.46)
% Cognitive Impairment	14.72	10.22	13.06	11.15	10.18
	(14.00)	(9.40)	(10.06)	(11.71)	(14.20)
% Behavior Problems	1.67	0.45	0.46	1.53	0.51
	(6.99)	(1.64)	(1.37)	(5.89)	(1.88)
% Physical Functioning	36.18	26.60	31.20	16.08	25.18
	(23.31)	(17.00)	(14.58)	(14.22)	(18.32)
Continuing Case Mix	(n = 366)	(n = 122)	(n = 142)	(n = 759)	(n = 94)
% Rehabilitation	2.71	2.19	0.85	1.18	1.51
	(5.79)	(7.57)	(1.41)	(1.94)	(2.11)
% Extensive	0.50	0.92	1.45	1.26	0.74
	(0.78)	(2.10)	(2.04)	(2.22)	(0.92)
% Special Care	4.28	5.17	11.11	9.42	5.11
	(2.96)	(3.13)	(6.00)	(6.46)	(2.68)
% Clinically Complex Care	30.64	34.11	32.46	40.72	38.03
	(12.20)	(9.05)	(8.21)	(10.74)	(7.82)
% Cognitive Impairment	16.52	13.33	13.66	12.67	11.55
	(7.24)	(7.22)	(5.82)	(7.00)	(4.86)
% Behavior Problems	2.35	1.05	0.97	2.32	1.16
	(7.41)	(1.44)	(1.65)	(4.07)	(1.51)
% Physical Functioning	43.00	43.23	39.49	32.44	41.89
	(13.15)	(10.63)	(8.35)	(10.85)	(9.08)

Value inside the parentheses is the standard distribution.

TABLE 2. Facility and Market Area Characteristics Calendar Year 1995–Free-standing Facilities Only

Characteristics	Kansas (n = 366)	Maine (n = 122)	Mississippi (n = 142)	Ohio (n = 759)	South Dakota (n = 94)
Facility Attributes					
Number beds in facility	75.51	73.06	103.20	106.80	72.99
	(36.42)	(37.81)	(50.97)	(63.46)	(32.56)
% NF's that are for profit facilities	48.09	82.00	89.40	79.40	41.50
% NF's that are in corporate chains	55.46	48.40	62.00	50.50	60.60
NF–SNF licensed (%)	51.64	100.0	57.00	69.00	57.40
Average age of NF residents	82.25	81.87	80.78	79.59	83.34
	(5.64)	(6.46)	(4.37)	(6.69)	(2.56)
% Facility residents on Medicaid	46.12	69.20	67.71	66.58	50.36
	(18.19)	(17.20)	(18.55)	(20.52)	(12.92)
Facility occupancy rate	84.92	93.06	95.26	85.57	95.54
	(16.74)	(6.81)	(8.78)	(17.18)	(4.61)
Service Demand					
% Aged 65+ in county	16.73	14.05	12.98	13.67	17.55
	(4.64)	(1.37)	(2.14)	(2.16)	(4.96)
% County females in labor force	52.47	53.67	45.81	50.47	53.32
	(5.85)	(4.27)	(6.20)	(5.46)	(7.41)
Per capita income (000s)	$19.78	$19.89	$16.30	$21.73	$18.73
	(3.92)	(3.19)	(2.65)	(3.77)	(3.32)
Hospital discharges per 1000 population	119.49	127.10	158.90	123.70	116.6
	(61.96)	(41.99)	(101.90)	(63.11)	(90.62)
Population/sq. mile in (000s)	0.15	0.13	0.10	0.87	0.031
	(0.26)	(0.107)	(0.09)	(0.97)	(0.049)
% County NF residents w/Medicare payment	14.19	12.50	7.83	16.68	37.31
	(9.42)	(2.93)	(5.08)	(6.83)	(7.76)
% County NF Residents w/Medicaid payment	45.08	66.76	65.70	65.11	50.67
	(8.05)	(6.59)	(12.51)	(6.83)	(8.47)
Service Supply					
Nursing facility beds per 1000 population	17.73	8.10	7.35	9.85	17.47
	(14.43)	(1.76)	(2.56)	(3.39)	(8.95)
Nursing facility residents per 1000 age 65+	87.61	62.43	58.30	61.47	108.20
	(63.49)	(13.70)	(17.6)	(34.83)	(38.51)
# RCF beds per 1000 county population	1.94	3.92	1.11	1.70	1.43
	(1.84)	(1.81)	(1.26)	(6.00)	(1.61)

Value inside the parentheses is the standard deviation. RCF refers to residential care facility, NF to nursing facility. All data are for 1995 other than % Females in the labor force (1990) and hospital discharge rates (1993).

Simulation analyses (reported in depth in Swan & Newcomer, in press) were used to partially overcome the empirical limitation of having only one year of observations and the constrained set of state policies and other conditions. The policies simulated were requiring that all nursing homes be licensed as skilled nursing facilities and that the supply of RCFs per 1000 population was set to the levels present in Maine in 1995. Simulation results suggest that nursing facility case mix, as expressed by the proportion of people with physical or cognitive impairment, could be reduced at time of *admission* by adoption of policies that restrict nursing home operations to skilled levels of care. The magnitude of this effect, though small in absolute terms (i.e., 1 to 4%), suggested relatively large proportionate reductions (i.e., 10% to 30% combining both cognitive and physical RUG classified cases) among the target case mix categories. This reduction was most substantial in a state with relatively lower observed proportions of patients in the physical problem or cognitively impaired case mix groups, suggesting that the simulated policies supplemented other existing nursing home utilization policies. In most states the effect was more evident in reference to the cognitively impaired. These effects were generally not enhanced under the assumption of an expanded RCF supply. This was true even for states having either facilitative RCF reimbursement or RCF eligibility criteria.

Among the *continuing* population, the simulated SNF policy had very little effect on either physical or cognitive problem case mix within any of the states. The simulated condition of expanded RCF supply, however, did suggest a minor reduction (about a 1% absolute change, about 10% in relative terms) in most of the states, and for both groups of conditions.

CONCLUSIONS

Together, the basic analyses and the simulations raise caution about the optimistic assumptions of the interplay between RCF policy and nursing home use. First, the upper limit of the proportion of nursing home cases with only physical and cognitive impairment likely to be affected by current and emerging long term care policy appears to be well under 35% of the current nursing home population–perhaps more in the range of a 10% to 20% reduction from among the prevailing number of cognitively or physical problem cases. This is suggested both by the simulation and the observed RUG rates. Further, the findings suggest that particular attention be given to continuing nursing home residents and the factors influencing the retention of cases with predominately physical or cognitive impairments. These proportions are more similar among states than case mix at admission, and they do not appear to have much association with RCF supply.

Additionally, there is the issue of supply and demand and how they interact. As state policy and other circumstances begin to alter the presumed balance between the demand for and supply of long-term services, the direction of adjustment in terms of bed supply and case mix may prove to be unpredictable. This unpredictability may not favor state Medicaid budgets if nursing home use does not change. For example, communities with more constrained nursing home supply may be in the status of having a level of demand that exceeds supply. If providers (in this context either nursing facilities or RCFs) are able to attract higher-paying residents, state policies that alter the demand for other long term care services are likely to have little impact on nursing home utilization until the supply of both nursing homes and RCFs catches up with the latent demand. The analyses suggest that while the excess demand may be more likely to use RCFs as they are available, there continues to be sufficient demand to keep nursing home use relatively stable. This finding is consistent with an analysis of continuing care retirement communities, which found that the presence of assisted living beds was associated with reduced days in independent living, not reduced nursing home days (Newcomer, Preston, Roderick, 1995). Of the states included in this analysis, Ohio is the most interesting. This state seems to have policies in place that are relatively effective in constrained access to nursing homes, yet the simulation results suggested even further reductions in the presence of increased RCF supply.

Conclusions drawn from these findings are qualified. The foremost limitation is that while nursing home demand was estimated, reductions in nursing home supply were simulated only by requiring them to be licensed for skilled care. Reductions in bed supply could substantially alter the demand for beds by each of the RUG classifications.

Important too is the existing disparity between the number of nursing home beds per 1000 population and that of RCF beds in most of the study states. Within Maine, the reference case for the simulations, the ratio was essentially 2:1 (i.e., 8.1 nursing home beds vs. 3.9 RCF beds per 1000 population). In the other four states the ratio of nursing beds to RCFs was much higher: South Dakota 12:1, Kansas 9:1, Mississippi 7:1, and Ohio 6:1. A related issue is that nursing home demand/use within a county (particularly those in rural areas) can be influenced by factors external to the county. These include bed availability in emigrant counties, and the relative difference in access to hospital and medical assistance and the presence of family or community resources between the sending and receiving counties. In states, such as Kansas, with a relatively high supply of nursing home beds in some counties, the demand for nursing homes may be more affected by a growth of RCF supply in the feeder communities than in the county where the nursing home is located.

A third caution is that the attainment of a balanced supply mix is not sufficient to explain case mix. Presently, Maine, Ohio, and Mississippi (each with different nursing home and RCF supplies) have similar numbers of nursing home residents per 1000 aged and similar proportions of cognitively impaired RUG classified cases in nursing homes. They vary only in the proportion classified with physical problems. This suggests that other nursing home utilization controls affecting nursing home case mix may be operating that were not directly measured.

A more problematic limitation in the study and the simulations is that facilitative RCF reimbursement policy was constrained below market housing rates by the empirically limited options available within the study states. Publicly subsidized RCF reimbursement comparable to market rates could likely reduce a larger proportion of nursing home residents for whom Medicaid is the primary payer than was estimated here. However, on average, the proportion of Medicaid patients would have to be reduced by 50% to effect a 25% reduction in the total number of nursing home patients.

Finally, it is important to note that all preexisting state utilization controls and other policies affecting nursing home placement and retention have been held constant in these analyses. This has been necessitated by the limit of five states in the current sample, and the confounding of various policies typically occurring in combination within some states. A logical extension of the current work would be an in-depth analysis of those states already having low proportions of nursing home patients in physically and cognitively impaired RUG classifications. Such analyses become feasible as more states have operational MDS data files, or within the same state over time.

REFERENCES

Fries, B.F., Schneider, D.P., Foley, W.J., Gavazzi, M., Burke, R., & Cornelius, E. (1994). Refining a case-mix measure for nursing homes: Resource utilization groups (RUG-III). *Medical Care, 32* (7): 668-685.

Mollica, R.L. (1998). *State Assisted Living Policy: 1998.* Portland, ME: National Academy of State Health Policy.

Newcomer, R., Preston, S., & Roderick, S. (1995). Assisted living and nursing unit use among continuing care retirement community residents. *Research on Aging, 17* (2): 149-167.

Newcomer, R., Swan, J., Bigelow, W., Harrington, C., Zimmerman, D., & Karon, S. (1999). Residential care supply and the cognitive and physical problem case mix among nursing facility residents. (A report to the Commonwealth Fund under grant number 96611.) San Francisco: University of California.

Spector, W., Reschovsky, J., & Cohen, J. (1996). Appropriate placement of nursing homes residents in lower levels of care. *Milbank Quarterly, 74* (1): 139+.

Swan, J., & Newcomer, R. (1999). A simulation of the effects of nursing home licensing policy and residential care supply on nursing home case mix. *Health Care Financing Review, 21* (3): 1-27.

Chapter 5

Impacts of Profit Status
of Assisted Living Facilities

Wendy P. Crook
Linda Vinton

SUMMARY. Florida is a bellwether state in terms of the need for assisted living among elderly persons and has more than 2,000 of the nation's estimated 11,459 assisted living facilities (ALFs). The authors of this article surveyed 140 ALFs in Florida in order to examine the relationship of profit status to ownership of other facilities, willingness to serve low income groups, formal policies, and persons involved in decisions about resident retention. Significant differences were found between for-profit and non-profit facilities in terms of ownership of nursing homes and resident involvement in retention decisions. A discussion of how the profit motive and formal policies can impact residents concludes the article. *[Article copies available for a fee from The Haworth Document Delivery Service: 1-800-342-9678. E-mail address: <getinfo@haworthpressinc.com> Website: <http://www.HaworthPress.com> © 2001 by The Haworth Press, Inc. All rights reserved.]*

KEYWORDS. Assisted living facilities, homes for the aging, organizations

Wendy P. Crook, PhD, is Assistant Professor, Florida State University, School of Social Work, Tallahassee, FL 32306-2570. Linda Vinton, PhD, is Associate Professor, Florida State University, School of Social Work, Pepper Institute on Aging and Public Policy, Tallahassee, FL 32306-2570.

[Haworth co-indexing entry note]: "Chapter 5. Impacts of Profit Status of Assisted Living Facilities." Crook, Wendy P., and Linda Vinton. Co-published simultaneously in *Journal of Housing for the Elderly* (The Haworth Press, Inc.) Vol. 15, No. 1/2, 2001, pp. 67-78; and: *Assisted Living: Sobering Realities* (ed: Benyamin Schwarz) The Haworth Press, Inc., 2001, pp. 67-78. Single or multiple copies of this article are available for a fee from The Haworth Document Delivery Service [1-800-342-9678, 9:00 a.m. - 5:00 p.m. (EST). E-mail address: getinfo@haworthpressinc.com].

INTRODUCTION

Home-based options for individuals who require varying degrees of long-term care are expanding but, according to The Institute for Health & Aging (1996):

> Today, many people who have lost or never acquired the ability to perform basic tasks of daily living receive care through a system that simply does not help them enough. Thousands of health care and social service programs . . . and several financing options . . . are already in place nationwide. Despite these efforts, many people with chronic conditions need, but are not getting, help with the elementary tasks of personal care and living in a complex world. (p. 56)

Not getting the help one needs leaves individuals at risk of injury and diminished quality of life. Mor and Allen (1994) investigated the personal consequences of unmet need by studying a random sample of persons with disabilities in Springfield, Massachusetts. Among the elders in the sample, 60% said they had not bathed or showered due to fear of falling; 58% reported not getting to the bathroom or changing often enough; 58% had experienced a fall when transferring; 29% had missed a medical appointment; and 25% had been unable to fill prescriptions or buy medical supplies when needed.

Assisted living is a community-based long-term care option that was initially developed to help disabled adults with everyday living. While many young and middle-aged adults require various types of supportive housing, the need for daily assistance among frail elderly persons, in particular, has spurred the growth of the assisted-living industry. Assisted living has been defined by Kane and Wilson (1993) as "any group residential program that is not licensed as a nursing home, that provides personal care to persons with need for assistance in the activities of daily living, and that can respond to unscheduled needs for assistance that might arise" (p. xi). The latter part of this definition suggests that supportive services will be available 24 hours a day. This aspect is found in all of the definitions of assisted living used by the various professional associations, American Association of Retired Persons, and U.S. Health Care Financing Administration. Two commonly stated purposes of assisted living are to maximize the individual functioning and autonomy of residents (Manard & Cameron, 1997) and to allow residents to age in place (Mollica, 1998).

Data from a survey of a nationally representative sample of assisted-living facilities (ALFs) estimated that there are 11,459 ALFs in the U.S. (Hawes, Rose, & Phillips, 1999). More than 2,000 of those facilities (with more than 70,000 beds) were in Florida alone. Florida's ALF facilities are highly diverse in terms of size, location, amenities, and cost. With the median age and proportion of elderly residents in year 2000 already at the levels that are expected nationwide by 2010, Florida is a bellwether state (U.S. Bureau of the Census, 1989). This article describes an empirical study of ALFs in Florida that examined relationships among organizational variables.

Following an earlier assisted-living policy synthesis, the Lewin-VHI, Inc. group (1996) prepared a literature review on assisted living for the frail elderly for the Administration on Aging and U.S. Department of Health and Human Services. They reported that between 1992 and 1995, the source of almost two-thirds of the literature on assisted living was provider or other trade publications (47%) and reports by associations, public policy think tanks, and consulting firms (18%). Only 17 articles or 10% of the literature described empirical research, and these studies were predominately descriptive, lacking conceptualization, and limited by the use of convenience samples. In contrast, the research discussed in this article had an explanatory purpose and used organizational concepts, systematic sampling, and bivariate analyses to answer whether profit status of ALFs was associated with ownership of other facilities, willingness to serve low income groups, formal policies, degree of bureaucracy, and persons involved in decision making about resident retention.

LITERATURE REVIEW

In an examination of states' assisted living policies, Mollica (1998) found 14 different terms used for assisted living (assisted living facilities/homes/residences, residential long term/care facilities, personal care boarding homes, shelter care facilities, supported residential living/care facilities, community based residential facilities, homes for the aged, large group/adult care homes, board and lodging, registered housing with services, comprehensive personal care homes, enriched housing programs, residences for adults, basic care facilities, and boarding homes). Florida uses the term "assisted living facility" and defines it as any residence, whether for-profit or not, that undertakes through its ownership or management to provide housing, meals, and one or more personal services for a period exceeding 24 hours to one or more adults who are not relatives of the owner or administrator (F.S. 400.402). This definition is similar to the eligibility criteria used in a recent national survey of facilities (Hawes, Rose, & Phillips, 1999). In that study, facilities were sampled that had more than 10 beds, served a primarily elderly population, and either represented themselves as assisted living facilities or offered at least a basic level of services that included 24 hour staff oversight, housekeeping, at least two meals a day, and some type of personal assistance (p. E-2).

Who lives in ALFs may be dictated not only by the older person's service needs and what type of care the facility offers, but also by state regulations (e.g., license type and level of care standards) and the residents' and/or residents' family members' ability to pay. Kane and Wilson (1993) conducted a national study of assisted living with a sample of 63 ALF administrators (65%

of the ALFs represented were for-profit and 35% non-profit). In terms of residents' need for assistance, they found that 25% of the residents sampled had what they characterized as low need, 50% had a medium need, and 25% had a high need for assistance.

Coopers Lybrand (1993) surveyed 201 assisted living providers in 25 states (75% of the ALFs were for-profit, 21% non-profit, and 4% publicly held) for the Assisted Living Facilities Association of America. In that study, ALF residents had a mean number of 3.06 activities of daily living (ADL) impairments and 42% were cognitively impaired to some degree. The typical resident was said to need "moderate or heavy care." In comparison, the Florida Policy Exchange Center on Aging and Southeast Florida Center on Aging (1996) surveyed a randomly drawn statewide sample of assisted living residents aged 60 and older (N = 736) in Florida and reported somewhat lower levels of impairment. The mean number of non-independent ADLs for the Florida sample was 2.13 and 21% had severe cognitive impairment (41% of the residents, though, were noted to have some type of dementia). These studies imply that residents have varying levels of need for services available through the ALF model.

As noted above, the purpose of assisted living is generally to allow impaired elders to age in place. This concept or philosophy is not a guarantee, however. Hawes, Rose, and Phillips (1999) found that ALF services did not always match the philosophy of assisted living. For instance, in some facilities, retention policies meant that a resident could reasonably expect to live to the end of his or her life in the facility regardless of physical or cognitive decline; whereas in others, "aging in place" was a qualified term and a change in needs could mean that the resident would be discharged.

ORGANIZATIONAL FACTORS

According to Brager and Holloway (1978), human service organizations are ". . . formal organizations that have as their stated purpose enhancement of the social, emotional, physical, and/or intellectual well-being of some component of the population" (p. 2). Thus, assisted living facilities may be considered human service organizations. Similar to the purpose of human service organizations in general, the key tenets of the philosophical underpinnings of assisted living are policies that emphasize dignity, autonomy, and services that enhance independence and aging in place (Hawes, Rose, & Phillips, 1999).

In recent years, the direct-service role of the public sector has declined. The number of for-profit companies that offer services typically provided by non-profit and government organizations has increased (Gibelman, 2000). However, the efficacy of this trend has been questioned on two fronts: overall efficiency and impacts on clients. There is little evidence to date that shows that privatized human services are more efficient and lead to better outcomes for clients than not-for-profit agency services. A focus on profitability can produce aggressive marketing and pricing strategies in order to achieve financial gain, with the result being a decline in clients' quality of care (Gibelman, 2000). This is relevant to the ALF industry because proprietary firms have proliferated in the long-term care sector (Netting, Kettner, & McMurtry, 1993).

Bureaucracy refers to an organizational form characterized by hierarchy based on authority, division of labor, and procedures and rules. Bureaucracies are designed for efficiency and reliability (Hall, 1982). The formalization that characterizes bureaucratic organizations is used to standardize decision-making among organizational members by requiring them to follow administratively-established policies and procedures. In terms of formal policies in ALFs, Mollica (1998) reported primarily on state rather than organizational level policies. Some states regulate the promulgation, posting, or distribution of rules in ALFs. Mollica categorized such policies as relating to general, health related, functional, dementia, and behavioral issues. Examples of organizational policies would be admission, retention, and discharge guidelines that pertain to all residents. Health, functional, dementia, and behavioral policies may apply to some but not all residents and put limits on the types and amounts of physical and/or mental health care facilities can offer.

Kane and Wilson (1993) examined policies and practices relating to resident choice. They labeled these policies as autonomy-enhancing. Pet ownership, visiting hours, overnight guests, smoking, alcohol use, seating at meals, access to residents' rooms, the right to refuse service, resident governance, medication management, and transportation were the areas that Kane and Wilson asked respondents to comment on in their survey of ALFs. They found about 40% of the settings allowed pets; 75% had flexible visiting hours and allowed guests either in the resident's or guest room; half allowed smoking in designated areas (one-third in residents' rooms); almost half had a seating assignment policy; 40% said they required staff to knock before entering residents' rooms; 79% had resident governance procedures or councils; and 88% offered transportation as a service. The right to refuse services varied, but only 14% reported it was the resident's choice to refuse, and ambiguous or complex policies on medication management did not allow the authors to do an analysis.

Profit and ownership status and policies and services have been found to vary among ALFs (Hawes, Rose, & Phillips, 1999). Other organizational characteristics such as degree of bureaucracy and persons involved in "aging in place" decisions have not been studied. Furthermore, the relationships between these variables has not been explored, along with their relationship to resident outcomes. The following conceptual model was employed in the study described herein (see Figure 1).

FIGURE 1. Conceptual Model

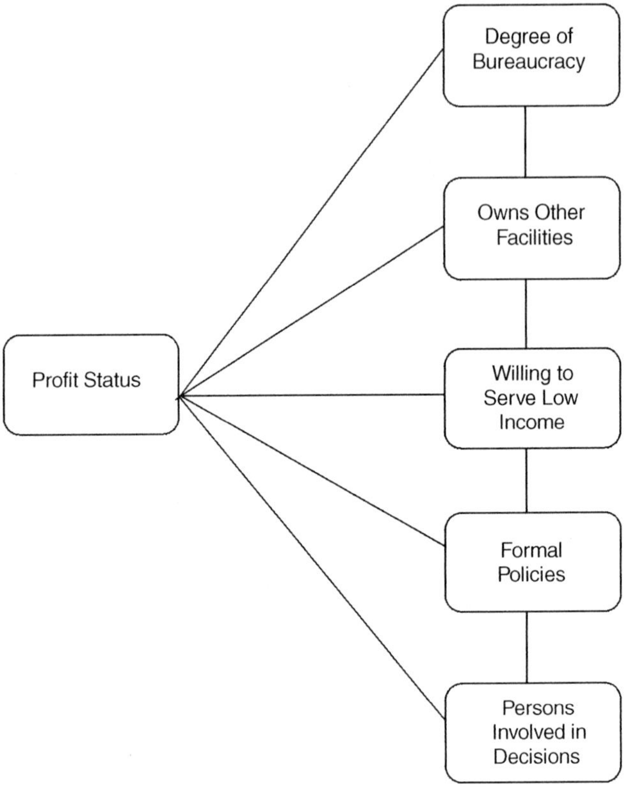

METHODOLOGY

A survey design was employed to solicit information about the organizational characteristics of ALFs. The sample was derived from a 1997 Florida Agency for Health Care Administration listing of licensed ALFs. Systematic sampling was used to select every fifth ALF for a total of 366 facilities. This sample was augmented with the remaining number of ALFs that were enrolled providers of ALF Medicaid Waiver services (n = 73) in order to ensure that non-profit facilities were represented in the sample.

The survey questionnaire was designed by the researchers and pilot tested with 20 ALF administrators whose facilities were not selected for the study. After revisions were made, the final survey was mailed to the attention of ALF administrators. A second mailing was done in order to increase the response rate. The questionnaire contained a combination of forced-choice and open-ended questions. Twenty-six questions explored characteristics of the facility, such as size, auspice, types of formal policies, degree of bureaucracy, and decision making processes. Descriptive statistics were used and chi-square analyses were performed in order to examine relationships between for profit status and degree of bureaucracy and ownership of other facilities, willingness to serve low income groups, formal policies, and persons involved in decision making about resident retention.

RESULTS

Description of the Respondent ALFs

Among the 439 questionnaires that were mailed, 10 were undeliverable and 140 were returned, thus yielding a 33% response rate. ALF administrators reported having between 3 and 394 beds in their facilities ($\overline{x} = 49$) with approximately half having 20 or fewer and half more than 20 beds. The mean occupancy rate was 82% with slightly more than two-thirds saying their rate was 75% or higher.

The majority of ALFs offered meals, housekeeping, activities, 24 hour supervision, laundry service, medication management, assistance with ADLs, medical and non-medical transportation, and cable television in their basic rate. Less than a majority offered personal care (47%) and nursing services (42%), and only 15% provided adult incontinency supplies. A small number of respondents reported covering other services in the basic rate, such as physical therapy, companionship, telephones, movies, and dining out.

The average lowest monthly rates for the ALFs in the sample ranged from $337 to $2,500 with a mean of $1,004 (mode was $612 which coincided with Florida's Supplemental Security Income [SSI] amount). Average highest monthly rates ranged from $504 to $4,500, with a mean of $1,681. Since the sample was augmented with facilities that accepted Medicaid, average rates were likely skewed lower. By way of comparison, national data on assisted living facilities with a single rate yielded an average monthly rate of $1,710 (range $300-$6,400) and for facilities with multiple rates, the average monthly rate was $1,582 (range $300-$7,130) (Hawes, Rose, & Phillips, 1999).

Description of Organizational Characteristics

The vast majority of respondents said their ALFs were for-profit (84%). For approximately one-third, the ALF was their only facility. Among those respondents that said they or their owners had other facilities, 21% reported owning at least one skilled nursing facility. Slightly more than half of the sample said they accepted low income residents or individuals who received SSI along with the state's board and care supplement.

Formalization was examined by asking ALF administrators about the degree of bureaucracy in their organizations, whether they had developed written policies, and the frequency of involving certain persons in decisions about residents. Two-thirds of the administrators said the degree of bureaucracy was medium to high in their organizations, and one-third said there was either no or a low degree of bureaucracy. The vast majority of respondents had written policies concerning personnel (92%), admissions (91%), discharge (89%), and resident safety (87%), and most had policies about behavior management (71%) and incontinency (63%).

With respect to the parties that are involved in making decisions about whether residents can "age in place" at the ALF or whether they need to be transferred, more than three-fourths of the respondents said they always involve the resident's physician, administrator, and family members. Approximately half always involved the ALF owner and residents themselves (Figure 2).

Bivariate Analyses

Bivariate relationships were examined between for-profit status and five variables: ownership of other facilities; willingness to serve low income

FIGURE 2. Percent of Respondents Stating Persons Always Involved in Decision Making Concerning Resident Retention (Aging in Place)

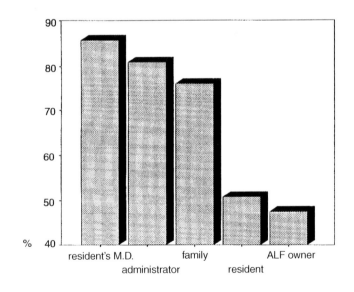

groups; formal policies; degree of bureaucracy; and people involved in resident retention decisions. Interestingly, non-profit ALFs were significantly
more likely to say they or their owners also owned skilled nursing facilities
(47%) than for-profit ALFs (22%) (p = .047). And while it might be expected
that the non-profit ALFs would be more likely to accept low income residents,
no difference was seen between the groups; 55% of the for-profit respondents
and 60% of the non-profit ALFs stated they would accept persons on SSI along
with the state board and care supplement. For-profit and non-profit ALFs were
also just as likely to have each type of formal policy (personnel, admission,
discharge, resident safety, behavior management, and incontinency policies),
and identical proportions (75%) of the profit and non-profit respondents said
their organizations had medium to high degrees of bureaucracy.

There was a significant difference between for-profit and non-profit ALFs
in terms of always involving residents in decisions about retention. More than
three-fourths (79%) of the non-profits always involved the resident in such decisions; whereas, only half (50%) of the for-profits always involved the residents (p = .05) (Figure 3).

The relationship between degree of bureaucracy and persons involved in
decision making was also examined but no significant differences were found.
Degree of bureaucracy, however, was found to be associated with two types of

FIGURE 3. Percent of Respondents Stating Persons Always Involved in Decision Making Concerning Resident Retention (Aging in Place) by Profit Status

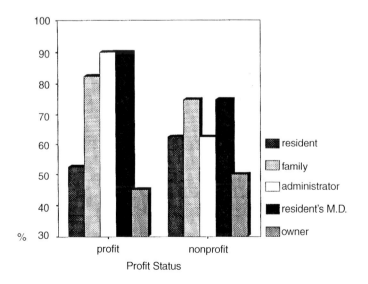

formal policy. ALFs reported to have a medium to high degree of bureaucracy were significantly more likely to have policies dealing with resident incontinency and behavior management than those reporting no to low bureaucracy. Almost three-fourths (74%) of the medium to high degree of bureaucracy ALFs had an incontinency policy versus 53% of the no to low degree of bureaucracy facilities (p = .023). Similarly, a high proportion of the medium to high degree of bureaucracy ALFs had behavior management policies (83%) as compared with 60% of the no to low degree of bureaucracy ALFs (p = .009).

DISCUSSION

The trade literature has taken note of the rapid growth of the assisted-living industry, and the empirical literature needs to follow. This study was explanatory and conceptualized assisted-living facilities as organizations. Although the study had sampling limitations, the respondents were diverse in terms of types of facilities that were represented in the sample. Consistent with other studies (Coopers Lybrand, 1993; Kane & Wilson, 1993), the ALF respondents in this study predominantly operated for-profit facilities.

The ALF administrators reported medium to high levels of bureaucracy, and most had written policies for incontinency and behavior management, thus indicating a high level of formalization regarding these particular resident control issues. The amount of formalization in an organization can be an indication of the perceptions of decision-makers regarding the ability of members to exercise judgement (Hall, 1982). Furthermore, while most of the facilities reported that non-ALF individuals (i.e., the resident's physician and/or family members) participate in decisions about the resident's status, only one-third or less always involve the resident him/herself. This is problematic, for "the exercise of discretion permits the service providers, while attending to the needs of clients, to make decisions that promote their own interests, which may not be consonant with those of the client" (Hasenfeld, 1983, p. 183). The basic right of self-determination is abrogated for residents in those facilities that are highly formalized and do not include the resident in decisions about her/his status, especially in the for-profit facilities, which involved the resident in retention decisions less than the non-profit facilities.

The profit motive may supercede the needs of residents in these for-profit organizations. Non-profit ALFs may involve residents in retention decisions more often than for-profit facilities because they are governed by voluntary Boards of Directors whose members are responsive to community norms. In terms of philosophy or governing principles, such facilities may also be more "client-centered" than for-profit ALFs.

Non-profit ALFs were affiliated with skilled nursing facilities significantly more often than for-profits. This may be a harbinger of a trend wherein nonprofits create hybrid organizations in order to successfully compete with for-profits in the long-term care marketplace. Further study in this area is needed, especially investigations focusing on the impact of such hybrid organizations on client outcomes.

More studies of the organizational characteristics of ALFs are needed that examine a wider range of impacts on residents. Many elders move to assisted facilities with the expectation that they can age (and even die) in place. This study found that organizational factors influenced whether facilities allowed residents to age in place. Such factors may be associated with other outcomes that affect resident well-being as well as peace of mind for residents' family members.

REFERENCES

Assisted Living Facilities, Florida Statutes §§ 400.402 (1999).

Brager, G., & Holloway, S. (1978). *Changing human service organizations: Politics and practice*. New York: Free Press.

Coopers & Lybrand. (1993). *An overview of the assisted living industry*. The Assisted Living Facilities Association of America.

The Florida Policy Exchange Center on Aging & The Southeast Florida Center on Aging. (June 1996). *Project Two: The Florida Long-Term Care Elder Population Profiles Survey*. Final Report to the Commission on Long-Term Care in Florida.

Gibelman, M. (2000). Structural and fiscal characteristics of social service agencies. In R. J. Patti (Ed.), *The handbook of social welfare management* (pp. 113-131). Thousand Oaks, CA: Sage.

Hall, R. H. (1982). *Organizations: Structure and process*. Englewood Cliffs, NJ: Prentice-Hall.

Hasenfeld, Y. (1983). *Human service organizations*. Englewood Cliffs: Prentice-Hall, Inc.

Hawes, C., Rose, M., & Phillips, C. D. (1999). *A national study of assisted living for the frail elderly*. Beachwood, OH: Myers Research Institute Menorah Park Center for Senior Living.

The Institute for Health & Aging. (August 1996). *Chronic care in America: A 21st century challenge*. Report prepared for The Robert Wood Johnson Foundation. San Francisco, CA: University of California.

Kane, R. A., & Wilson, K. B. (1993). *Assisted living in the United States: A new paradigm for residential care for frail older persons?* Washington, DC: American Association of Retired Persons.

Lewin-VHI, Inc. (February 1996). *National study of assisted living for the frail elderly: Literature review update*. Prepared for The Office of the Assistant Secretary for Planning and Evaluation and Administration on Aging, U.S. Department of Health and Human Services (HHS-100-94-0024). NC: Research Triangle Park.

Mollica, R. L. (1998). State assisted living policy: 1998 (DHHS-100-94-0024). Portland, ME: National Academy for State Health Policy.

Mor, V., & Allen, S. (1994). Unpublished results from the *Springfield, Massachusetts Study of populations with disabilities*. Providence, RI: Brown University.

Netting, F. E., Kettner, P. M., & McMurtry, S. L. (1993). *Social work macro practice.* White Plains, NY: Longman.

U.S. Bureau of the Census. (January 1989). Projections of the population of the United States, by age, sex, and race: 1988 to 2080 by Gregory Spencer. *Current Population Reports,* Series P-25, No. 1018. Washington, DC: Government Printing Office.

U.S. Bureau of the Census. (March 1997). *1992 Census of service industries, U.S. summary.* [Online]. Available: http://www.census.gov/epcd/www.sc92.html.

Chapter 6

A Framework for Understanding Homelike Character in the Context of Assisted Living Housing

John P. Marsden

SUMMARY. In the United States, assisted living has been promoted as a noninstitutional relocation choice offering personal care services for the elderly in a residential or homelike context. Yet, it is unknown whether assisted living, and, in particular, its exterior appearance, is actually perceived as homelike. Few researchers have addressed what home actually means in architectural terms to nontraditional populations such as the elderly, and even fewer have investigated homeyness in relation to assisted living. Drawing upon Grant McCracken's work, a framework is proposed which suggests that homeyness, in the context of the exterior appearance of assisted living, entails symbolic properties of

John P. Marsden, PhD, is Assistant Professor at Auburn University, 308 Spidle Hall, Auburn University, AL 36849. He holds a Bachelor of Architecture from Carnegie Mellon University, a Master of Architecture and Graduate Certificate in Gerontology from the University of Arizona, and a Master of Science and PhD in Architecture, with a minor in Gerontology, from the University of Michigan. This work was conducted under the direction of Rachel Kaplan and Kate Warner in partial fulfillment for a doctoral degree in architecture at the University of Michigan.

The author would like to thank Rachel Kaplan for her helpful contributions to this article.

[Haworth co-indexing entry note]: "Chapter 6. A Framework for Understanding Homelike Character in the Context of Assisted Living Housing." Marsden, John P. Co-published simultaneously in *Journal of Housing for the Elderly* (The Haworth Press, Inc.) Vol. 15, No. 1/2, 2001, pp. 79-96; and: *Assisted Living: Sobering Realities* (ed: Benyamin Schwarz) The Haworth Press, Inc., 2001, pp. 79-96. Single or multiple copies of this article are available for a fee from The Haworth Document Delivery Service [1-800-342-9678, 9:00 a.m. - 5:00 p.m. (EST). E-mail address: getinfo@haworthpressinc.com].

79

"supportive protection" as evidenced by familiar housing cues, enclosure, and care; "human scale"; and "naturalness." *[Article copies available for a fee from The Haworth Document Delivery Service: 1-800-342-9678. E-mail address: <getinfo@haworthpressinc.com> Website: <http://www.HaworthPress.com> © 2001 by The Haworth Press, Inc. All rights reserved.]*

KEYWORDS. Older adults, assisted living, homelike character

A house is a body like yours and mine. It's not such a stretch to think of beams as bones, electrical wiring as a nervous system, plaster and brick as the layers of skin that protect us from the elements. And yet uninhabited houses and bodies are only compelling to contractors and coroners. It takes a soul to give a body life. (Morgan, 1996, p. xiii)

The "soul" of housing is what homeyness is all about. As emphasized in the preceding quotation, home and housing, though sometimes used synonymously, are about very different concepts. Housing refers to a "bundle of services." One component is the physical unit or the collection of rooms occupying a certain amount of space and possessing certain features. The neighborhood environment consisting of social networks, physical characteristics, and natural amenities in which the physical unit exists is a second component. A third aspect includes the types, quantity, and quality of public services and utilities. The location of the physical unit from work, shopping, and other services is a fourth dimension, and a final component includes the economic investment of the unit and neighborhood (USCM and HUD, 1977). In contrast, "home is both a physical place *and* a cognitive concept" (Tognoli, 1987, p. 655). It refers to the dynamic combination of social, psychological, cultural, behavioral, and physical properties, which leads to an intangible, emotional, and sometimes even metaphysical relationship between the person and his or her housing. Many researchers have asserted that such a relationship distinguishes the concept of home from housing (Dovey, 1985; Saegert, 1985; Schwarz, 1999; van Vliet, 1998).

This notion of home is often of particular importance to the elderly who have relocated to a group living arrangement due to housing deficiencies, unavailable support, the loss of a partner, and/or physical and cognitive impairments. In the United States, assisted living, a relatively new housing option, claims to embrace the concept of home. It has been promoted as a noninstitutional relocation choice offering personal care services for the frail elderly in a residential or homelike context.

Yet, it is unknown whether assisted living, and, in particular, its exterior appearance, is actually perceived as homelike. This is largely due to gaps in the literature. For instance, the meaning of home has traditionally been studied in the context of the single-family house. This building type has dominated middle class consciousness as an ideal since the eighteenth century (Clark, 1986), and many people have experienced homeyness in that context. The meaning of home has also been explored primarily from the perspective of traditional households–middle-class married couples with young children living in owned single-family houses (Despres, 1991). Few have addressed what home actually means to nontraditional populations such as the elderly. As a result, research in the area of homeyness may not be applicable to settings such as assisted living which are larger and entail group living for seniors. In addition, physical properties that are thought to reinforce homelike character have received little empirical attention and have not been successfully integrated into theoretical perspectives (Despres, 1991; Moore, 2000). This makes it even more difficult to examine how homeyness can be communicated by buildings other than single-family houses. Moreover, most of the work in this area has not been supported by empirical evidence, and a conceptual framework to guide research is lacking in the field (Rapoport, 1985). This has prevented meaningful comparisons between different housing contexts, populations, and cultures.

The purpose of this article is to first provide an overview of the work that has been conducted by researchers hoping to gain an understanding of what home means to the elderly. This may, at the very least, provide glimpses of homeyness cues. The second section of the investigation identifies symbolic as well as physical properties of home and, in the process, offers a useful framework for studying the communication of homeyness in buildings in general. In a third section, a revised and more refined framework is proposed in relation to the exterior appearance of assisted living housing for the elderly.

AN OVERVIEW OF HOME FOR THE ELDERLY

A few researchers have explored the meaning of home as it pertains to the elderly (Boschetti, 1984; Dupuis and Thorns, 1996; Fogel, 1992; Howell, 1985; Norris-Baker and Scheidt, 1994; O'Bryant, 1983; Pastalan and Schwarz, 1993; Rowles, 1983, 1987; Rubinstein, 1989; Sixsmith and Sixsmith, 1991). This has involved an understanding of the interaction between people and the home environment in the context of the life experience as a whole. Although this literature is scant and only pertains to the elderly living in individual houses rather than in housing designated for seniors, several meanings of home have been identified based on descriptions from the elderly. Pastalan and Schwarz (1993) have provided the most complete compilation of those dimensions. These include: (a) home as a safe place which provides protection from outside threats and facilitates competence in a familiar environment, (b) home as the center of loving relationships with family, (c) home as a place of choice regarding lifestyle and activities, (d) home as a territory one controls through personalization, architectural appearance, furniture arrangement, and the monitoring of the ambient environment and behavior, (e) home as a reflection of personal identity, (f) home as a place that protects one's privacy, (g) home as a place of continuity or a connection to one's past, (h) home as an expression of social status or achievement through ownership and architectural appearance, and (i) home as a place where one prefers to die.

The meanings of home Pastalan and Schwarz (1993) identified for the elderly are nearly identical to categories Despres (1991) provided based on a comprehensive review of the literature on traditional households. Common themes are issues of control, privacy, territoriality, security, and ownership; the house as the center of loving relationships and activities; and the house as an expression of social status and personal identity both past and present. Only three differences are apparent. For the elderly, there is a greater emphasis on familiarity as a meaning of home. Over time, seniors often develop an inherent " 'body-awareness' of every detail of the physical configuration" of the home environment (Rowles, 1983, p. 302). They are familiar with how the house is ordered and with its contents. As a result, the environment becomes predictable and can be taken for granted. This familiarity can compensate for progressive sensory losses likely to accompany old age, can facilitate competence, can ensure security, and can help the elderly maintain mastery over the home range. There is also an emphasis on choice with respect to activities for the elderly. With advancing age, there are often physical, cognitive, and social losses that may impose restrictions and highlight the need for choice in other facets of an individual's life. One other apparent difference is that the elderly are more likely to consider the imminence of death. This is often a part of the everyday reality of the elderly and impacts long-term plans (Sixsmith and Sixsmith, 1991). For instance, relocating to a new place may seem futile despite impairments. This may be why home is described by Pastalan and Schwarz as a place where one prefers to die.

Despite the similar meanings provided by Despres (1991) for traditional households and by Pastalan and Schwarz (1993) for the elderly, the studies in both literature reviews generally neglect to consider the physical properties of single family houses which have shaped these meanings. For instance, to state that a house which provides a sense of security is homey is nebulous. Security presumably involves protecting occupants from the elements or outside intruders. Such a description does not, however, identify specific physical features or spatial relationships which would help to physically or psychologically create a sense of security. Despres (1991) found in reviewing the literature that the majority of investigations give priority to territorial behavior and an individual's psychological make-up, personal life experiences, and affiliation with different societal groups as forces which define the meaning of home. The impact of physical features of housing on people's perceptions, judgments, and experiences of home typically were not addressed. In addition, Despres asserted that these physical properties were rarely integrated into theoretical perspectives such as territorial behavior or psychological make-up.

Despres recommended reviewing studies outside mainstream Environment and Behavior research which may provide insights into the impact of physical features on the home experience. One such study which is relevant to an investigation of the exterior appearance of assisted living is an ethnographic research project conducted by anthropologist Grant McCracken (1989). His work is discussed in the next section.

McCRACKEN'S PROPERTIES OF HOMEYNESS

McCracken (1989) drew upon previous social science research, particularly in the areas of anthropology and consumer goods and behavior. He indicated that homeyness, in the context of the North American house, depends on an understanding of (a) the symbolic meanings which endow physical properties with "cultural significance" (p. 170) and (b) the ways that physical properties help make these symbolic meanings material. Unlike an image, which is a reproduction or imitation of an artifact and a sign which stands for something in a literal sense, symbolic meaning is the result of "a cognitive process whereby an environment acquires a connotation beyond its instrumental use" (Lang, 1987, p. 204) and arouses an association or emotion. Physical properties, according to McCracken (1989), include many aspects of the house, such as its "colors, materials, furniture, decorative objects, arrangement, interior design, and exterior characteristics" (p. 169). In other words, it refers to features of a dwelling which cannot be easily modified, such as size, layout, and aesthetic aspects as well as movable elements typically associated with personalization.

In order to get to the root of homeyness, McCracken (1989) interviewed 40 Canadian men and women for six hours each. All participants lived in freestanding houses and were Caucasian, Protestant, of British descent, third-generation Canadian, and married. Half were blue collar and half were managerial. Based on descriptions provided by the participants, McCracken identified seven symbolic properties and several physical properties as defining characteristics of homeyness in the house. For the purpose of this work, only physical features relevant to the exterior envelope of the house are addressed. The symbolic properties are discussed in relation to these physical properties.

   a. *The Diminutive Property* "makes an environment more graspable, conceivable, thinkable . . ." (p. 171). Front doors and windows are small, proportions are manageable, and roofs are low.
   b. *The Variable Property* "appears to deliberately eschew uniformity and consistency" (p. 171). There is a preference, for example, for houses made of rubble stone rather than cut stone.

c. *The Embracing Property* "demonstrates a descending pattern of enclosure. The structure of the neighborhood, the foliage of the street and yard, the ivy of the exterior wall, the overhanging roof, the exterior wall ... all work by graduated stages to create the sense of enclosure" (p. 172).

d. *The Engaging Property* "appears deliberately designed to engage the observer." For example, "the wreath has something in its character that extends an invitation for interaction, promises a warm reception, represents a certain emotional tone for the interior within" (p. 173).

e. *The Mnemonic Property* "has the effect of deeply personalizing the present circumstances" (p. 174). "Objects are intended to recall the presence of family and friendship relationships, personal achievements, family events, ritual passages, and community associations" (p. 173).

f. *The Authentic Property* makes "spaces and things" seem "more 'real' and somehow more 'natural' than certain alternatives . . . which are the product of modern aesthetics, interior designers, showpiece homes, and high status individuals" (p. 174).

g. *The Informal Property* entails warm colors such as orange, gold, brown, and green. The "exterior details of the house design are deliberately rustic, rural, cottage-like, and unprepossessing" (p. 174).

In addition, McCracken asserted that these properties may work in tandem. When the external wall consists of small (the diminutive property) and variable (the variable property) units such as brick and stone, for example, the surface is especially homey.

In contrast, many researchers focusing on homeyness, and in particular house exteriors, have investigated preferences for certain single-family house styles (Devlin, 1994; Duncan, 1973; Fusch and Ford, 1983; Langdon, 1982; Lansing, Marans, and Zehner, 1970; Nasar, 1993). Some have indicated that it is possible to make accurate inferences about a homeowner's personality based on exterior housing cues (Cherulnik and Wilderman, 1986; Sadalla, Verschure, and Burroughs, 1987; Werthman, 1968). A few others have also indicated that it is possible to make accurate inferences about a homeowner's occupation or social status based on exterior building appearance (Cherulnik and Wilderman, 1986; Royse, 1969), styles (Nasar, 1993; Werthman, 1968), building materials (Sadalla and Sheets, 1993), or landscape taste (Duncan, 1973). McCracken, however, approached homeyness as something which is "beyond style" (Kron, 1990, p. C1)–a concept which is more often understood by the formally educated. He addressed physical properties or the actual elements of style in single-family houses which symbolically reinforce homeyness. His properties may serve as a framework which can be used to investigate homeyness in other housing types. This is the subject of discussion in the next section.

PROPERTIES OF HOMEYNESS IN THE CONTEXT
OF ASSISTED LIVING

McCracken's (1989) symbolic and physical properties provide a framework for examining how homeyness can be communicated by single-family houses in North America. When this framework is viewed in relation to the *exterior* of a building type such as assisted living, however, some modification may be appropriate. Accordingly, a revised framework is proposed in light of McCracken's work and the other literature reviewed regarding the meaning of home. Specifically, the proposed framework focuses on three overarching themes: (1) "supportive protection" which encompasses three concepts, namely familiarity, enclosure, and care; (2) "human scale;; and (3) "naturalness." Each of these is discussed in turn along with physical properties which reinforce these symbolic themes.

Supportive Protection

Familiarity. McCracken indirectly addressed the concept of familiarity under the mnemonic property of homeyness when he indicated that personalization helps to recall family associations or achievements. In the context of assisted living housing, however, personalization to the exterior of the building is less pertinent. That does not belittle its importance; personalization is just more difficult to execute and examine in a group living arrangement. As a result, the mnemonic property is viewed somewhat differently. It is suggested that this property, through memory jogging symbols associated with the house, such as window shutters, may help to make an unfamiliar living arrangement more familiar for the elderly. Familiarity is a concept which was emphasized earlier in relation to the meanings of home identified by Pastalan and Schwarz (1993). The mnemonic property, viewed in this way, may provide a general sense of supportiveness, assurance, and protection.

In order to determine whether an environment is familiar, we relate current stimulation to memories of past experiences with environments. These experiences are stored as internal representations. Each representation is "a summary from a series of nonidentical experiences with a given object" (S. Kaplan and R. Kaplan, 1982, p. 26). In other words, this internal structure is not a copy or template of an environment; rather, it is an economical unit of knowledge consisting of the salient features of an environment. Familiarity results when characteristics of an environment have been frequently encountered before, and there is a fit between current stimulation and an existing internal representation. This can lead to a positive affective response. When current stimulation is largely discrepant from an internal representation, an environment is experienced as unfamiliar, and this experience can evoke a negative affective response (Purcell and Nasar, 1992).

A number of studies that have addressed housing for the elderly have stressed the importance of familiarity in the home environment (Pastalan and Schwarz, 1993; Rowles, 1983, 1987; Rubinstein, 1989). Küller (1988) demonstrated how a collective housing unit decorated in an old and familiar style provided a much better therapeutic environment for the elderly than a geriatric hospital. Several other researchers asserted that it is therapeutic to pattern long-term care settings for people with dementia after the houses many lived in previously (Brawley, 1997; Calkins, 1988; Cohen and Weisman, 1991; Zeisel, 1999). As Calkins (1988) wrote, "If an environment is familiar, they [people with dementia] are more likely to be able to understand, and therefore, cope with it" (p. 32). Regnier (1994), Regnier et al. (1995), Brummett (1997), and Hoglund and Ledewitz (1999), in their investigations of assisted living, indicated that designing with a familiar architectural language is important. Specifically, Regnier (1994) and Regnier et al. (1995) suggested using familiar residential materials such as brick, wood, and stone, wood windows as opposed to aluminum frame commercial windows, and a sloped roof rather than a flat one. In addition, Regnier (1994) recommended observing historical and regional references to features of housing stock. The porch of the typical Midwestern house and the low-slung roof of the California bungalow are examples. Wilson (1995) substantiated that assisted living should have "an architectural style that is commonly associated with places where people have lived" (p. 141). These are important considerations for the elderly especially after relocating to a new housing environment such as assisted living. Familiar cues are understandable and reassuring. They can also facilitate the relocation process.

Enclosure. The second way in which supportive protection can be symbolized is through enclosure. McCracken's (1989) embracing property stressed this concept. Enclosure has to do with "the dream of being sheltered and protected–the need to be inside *something* that motivates us all. Being inside a cave, inside a room, under a canopy, within a great domed enclosure, behind a fence, in an arena, on a balcony, or on a porch, all are conditions of enclosure which carry specific connotations" (Moore, Allen, and Lyndon, 1974, p. 143). With respect to the outdoors, Alexander et al. (1977) similarly asserted that one "usually looks for a tree to put his back against, a hollow in the ground, a natural cleft which will partly enclose and shelter him" (p. 521). This need for enclosure in order to feel safe and protected is certainly not new and can be traced historically.

Many early buildings hugged the earth like a bear cub's den, designed for protection against tornadoes as well as excesses of heat or cold. Ranch houses were designed for protection against enemies and the sun, with air circulation in mind; porches were added for sitting outside and as a center for observation and conviviality. Many vernacular houses represent a safe place, almost a fortress, a reflection of a basic tribal memory of the need for security, a need that modern man, beset by different enemies, feels as strongly as his forebears. (Kavanaugh, 1983, p. 13)

For the modern middle-class human, the single-family house was initially promoted as a refuge from the "instability of a transient society and the competitiveness of the business world." The post World War II era of suburban expansion reinforced "a feeling of protectiveness by using trees, lawns, and parks to create a pastoral-like setting. With its green lawns, and shade trees, nature itself was tamed and controlled in the suburbs" (Clark, 1986, p. 238).

A number of investigators, in addition to McCracken (1989), have referred to protection in this sense especially with respect to the roof of the single-family house. Frank Lloyd Wright (1954) indicated that he often provided a ground-hugging "broad protecting roof shelter" (p. 33) with large projecting eaves over the whole building to give the dwelling the "essential look" of shelter (p. 16). The roof overhangs also protected the walls, another enclosing element which affords protection. Rapoport (1969) asserted that the pitched roof as opposed to the flat roof is symbolic of shelter while Rand (cited in Alexander et al., 1977) found that people still find the pitched roof a powerful symbol of shelter even after being exposed to the flat roofs of the Modern Movement during the twentieth century. Alexander et al. (1977) stated that a roof must not only be large and visible, it must also include living quarters within its volume. According to Alexander et al., "the roof itself only shelters if it contains, embraces, covers, surrounds the process of living" (p. 570).

With respect to other features which symbolically reinforce the notion of protection in the house, Alexander et al. (1977) suggested that if windows in upper stories are smaller, one may feel a greater sense of enclosure and safety while occupying those upper floors. Window muntins as opposed to big areas of clear glass may also reassure the occupant that there is something enclosing him or her and providing protection. Bay windows suggest personal enclosure and imply protection as well. In addition, Alexander et al. (1997) noted that it is balconies with "half-open enclosures around them–columns, wooden slats, rose-covered trellises–which are used most" (p. 783). One other study which focused on non-residential buildings, a distinct difference from the studies cited thus far, found that articulated walls which produce variations in the depth of the facade and provide sheltered spaces are favored (Frewald, 1989). In addition, certain elements associated with the house such as front lawns or porches offer varying degrees of transition between the public street and the private house, and this is connected with protection (Alexander et al., 1977; Mugerauer, 1993).

While most researchers have investigated the notion of protection in the context of the single family house, two other studies, using open-ended case study approaches, addressed this symbolic property as it pertains to assisted living housing (Brummett, 1997; Regnier, 1994). Regnier (1994) found that elements such as sloped roofs, attached porches, chimneys, balconies, and dormers contribute to homeyness. This is due to their symbolic associations. The porch, covered patios, or balconies, for example, create a buffer from the outside world. In a similar vein, Brummett (1997) proposed that a layered building envelope with varying degrees of transition implies a sense of protection.

Care. The third concept related to supportive protection is care. An environment may express care directly through the act of building, "as in the meticulous gingerbread details in the little houses at Oak Bluff on Martha's Vineyard in Massachusetts" (Moore and Allen, 1976, p. 139). Brummett (1997) indicated that a fine level of detail and articulation can reflect care in the design of assisted living. Care, however, is probably most associated with maintaining or tending a place (Moore, Allen, and Lyndon, 1974). When landscaping is neat, fences are freshly painted, and details like window boxes or shutters are given attention, care is evident (Nassauer, 1995). This also suggests that there is a human presence. A person has been to that place and returns often (Nassauer, 1995). Signs of occupancy such as drawn curtains, open windows or outdoor seating also suggest human presence. Human presence, as demonstrated through occupancy and attention to details and maintenance, implies that support is nearby if needed. This may provide assurance for an elderly person who is likely to feel vulnerable if he or she is dealing with age-related losses and impairments.

Human Scale

A second theme labeled human scale is also proposed for the study of the exterior of assisted living housing in relation to McCracken's (1989) diminutive and engaging aspects of homeyness. For example, human scale, a significant dimension of the diminutive property, helps to make an environment more graspable and manageable. This is an important consideration for the elderly who may be experiencing age-related sensory, physical, or cognitive losses. An environment which is or appears more manageable may instill a sense of competence in the elderly. This type of environment is certainly more inviting. Thus, the diminutive property and the engaging property which stresses the welcoming aspect of homeyness can be addressed under the overarching theme of human scale.

What exactly is meant by human scale? This is not always entirely clear just as the concept of scale itself is often referenced in a variety of ways.

> We talk, for instance, of a large-scale housing development, and we usually mean just that it is big. In a different context, we say that an architectural drawing has a scale, meaning that so many units of measure on the drawing represent so many units of measure in the actual building. Then there are super scale, miniature scale, monumental scale, and–perhaps the most talked about of all–human scale. (Moore and Allen, p. 17)

One theme common to the various uses of the term scale is that the size of something is being compared to something else. For example, "a large scale development is large in comparison to an average housing development" (Moore and Allen, 1976, p. 17). That is not to say that scale is the same thing as size. Rather, "scale is *relative* size" (p. 18). Another commonality is that scale involves expectations based on past experiences (Orr, 1985). For instance, "super scale usually means that something is much bigger than we might have expected, miniature scale that it is much smaller" (Moore and Allen, 1976, pp. 17-18). Most things have a usual size which gives us a sense of how we should relate to them. A brick which is oversized, for example, will not meet our expectations and may seem disturbing as a result.

Human scale, then, suggests that something relates to the size of a human. A number of researchers have made reference to how the house relates to the human body in general. Bloomer and Moore (1977), for instance, described the single family house as "free-standing like ourselves, with a face and a back, a hearth (like a heart) and a chimney, an attic full of recollections of *up*, and a basement harboring implications of *down.* . . . There is generally a door like a mouth, windows like eyes, and a roof like a forehead, with symmetrical enhancements in front" (pp. 1-2). Cooper (1974), in a slightly different vein, suggested that the exterior of the house, like the outer layer of the body, represents the self we choose to display to others while the intimate interior is similar to the way we view ourselves. The detached single-family house as opposed to a high-rise apartment building also symbolizes our desire to be seen as separate, unique individuals. These studies, however, really refer to the human body as an ordering principle in relation to the single-family house.

Frank Lloyd Wright (1954) more closely addressed the idea of human scale by demonstrating how the body can serve as a measuring device in relation to the house. He stated that "human scale was true building scale" and used 5 feet 8 1/2 inches, his own height, "to fix every proportion of a dwelling or of anything in it" (p. 16). For instance, he eliminated "useless heights" or "empty grandeur" by lowering ceiling heights and roofs. The latter was accomplished by relocating servant quarters which were typically located in attic spaces in the earlier part of the twentieth century to rooms adjacent to the kitchen on the ground floor. Orr (1985) indicated that the spread of a human's arms, the length of a stride, and the size of a grip with one's hand in addition to human height are sources of human scale. A door knob which can be easily grasped especially if placed at a comfortable height from the ground, a brick which can be easily held with one hand, steps which have wide enough treads and risers within a certain range, and a doorway which is wide enough to pass through are examples. We cannot use these features easily unless they are related to the dimensions of the human body. With respect to the overall building, Orr (1985) asserted that greater attention to elements of a building which are large in relation to the body, rather than to smaller features such as doors, porch railings, or window muntins, tends to make a building appear monumental. In contrast, greater attention to smaller parts helps to create a feeling of intimacy or diminutiveness (Orr, 1985).

McCracken's engaging property which stresses the "welcoming" aspect of homeyness can also be included within the theme of human scale. This is because a building which emphasizes human scale is likely to be more manageable both visually and as a place to physically use. Orr (1985) referred to this notion when he stated that "a building should be almost huggable: it should present us with a surface or surfaces that we feel we could, if so inspired, physically embrace" (p. 54). Likewise, it appears that the building should, metaphorically, also open *itself* up, welcoming the observer and inviting entry in the process. Alexander et al. (1977) indicated that a glazed entry door can provide a glimpse of what is inside a building, alleviating any fears of the unknown and can allow the person approaching the building and those within to prepare for a reception. Thus, human scale can be more broadly interpreted as relating a building to the dimensions of the body in order to make it more manageable *and* welcoming.

This idea of human scale is particularly important when dealing with a housing type such as assisted living, which is larger than the single family house, and a group such as the elderly, who are typically more vulnerable than the general population. Robinson (1989), in her study of the differences between institutional housing and vernacular detached single-family housing, found that scale is a noticeable difference with respect to the building size and entrance approach. For instance, large institutional housing is usually set in expansive parklike grounds and includes a long formal entrance. Regnier et al. (1995), in their investigation of assisted living, offered recommendations for reducing scale in elderly housing. They stated that certain features such as porches, balconies, and dormers help to reduce the perceived mass and height of an assisted living building. Although they do not specifically refer to "human scale," they do stress that assisted living should "be perceived as small in size" (Regnier, 1994, p. 47). Similarly, Brummett (1997) proposed that an articulated building mass in both the wall plane through the creation of bays, clustering of units or creation of a base, and in the roof form through the use of dormers or changes in ridge lines, helps to relate the building to the individual. More specifically, he stated that window openings and panes, door openings, and finish materials and details should be of a "human-related size and refinement" (p. 49). In addition, Hoglund and Ledewitz (1999) stated that the building mass should be divided into smaller volumes to alleviate the monolithic character of many assisted living buildings.

Naturalness

McCracken's variable, authentic, and informal properties all appear to deal with the authentic or "real" quality of a place. These are combined in the proposed framework into a third theme, naturalness. Naturalness, as Frank Lloyd

Wright envisioned it, can be interpreted as close association to the natural environment by maximizing contact with the outdoors, using nature as a source of design inspiration for architectural forms and construction principles, heeding climatic conditions as they pertain to design, and using building materials in a way that is integral to the nature of the materials (Twombly, 1979). With respect to the exterior of buildings and the concept of homeyness, naturalness is largely related to landscape elements and the authentic use of building materials and color.

Nassauer (1995) reviewed a number of studies in the landscape perception literature which suggest that some landscape elements communicate naturalness. These studies have repeatedly identified elements such as vegetation, especially canopy trees, and water. S. Kaplan and R. Kaplan (1978, 1982), in their study of natural environments, suggested that certain landscape elements such as water and trees are considered desirable and enhance preference. The Kaplans contend that such preferred "contents" are linked to our evolutionary history and are interpreted as elements needed for survival. Nature itself is also a preferred content, and research has indicated that natural environments are preferred over both urban and residential environments (S. Kaplan, R. Kaplan, and Wendt, 1972).

Building materials can be considered modified elements of nature. Wood, for instance, was once alive. Although it doesn't continue to grow once it is cut down, it continues to remind us of its natural origins through its appearance, texture, and sometimes even its smell. The connection between materials and nature was particularly strong at one time.

> The materials from which a building was made came virtually from the site itself: stone was cut from local quarries and timber from neighboring forests; brick and tiles were baked in clay from nearby pits. There was a strong link between the artifact and the earth from which it grew that was not just economic, but deeply satisfying at a psychic level too. ("Materiality and Resistance," 1994, p. 4)

Color was also linked to nature. Often this was true because color is integral to specific building materials, such as red brick, and their weathering qualities. In addition, color was tied to specific regions and sites. "One of the most popular in New England–then and now–is red, which was applied on the exteriors of barns and houses to help absorb solar heat. In the days before paint was manufactured, New Englanders created a mixture of rust (scraped from nails and fences), skim milk, and lime that coated the wood like a varnish" (Kemp, 1987, p. 25).

This connection between materials, color, and nature was weakened "in the Industrial Revolution, when materials that had been common in one part of a country could be transported to another as whims of production and economics dictated" ("Materiality and Resistance," 1994, p. 4). While more traditional materials such as wood, brick, mud, straw, and plaster were tied to the site, processed, and put together by hand, buildings now are usually mass produced–built of factory-made, factory-finished materials. The connection between materials and nature was further weakened by the advent of modern materials and construction techniques. For instance, modern materials such as reinforced concrete, steel, plastic, imitation stone, and wood laminates are usually not perceived as "natural." "Steel is hard, cold, bearing the impress of the hard, powerful industrial machines that rolled or pressed it; plastic has something of the alien molecular technology of which it is made, standing outside the realm of life and, like reinforced concrete, bound by no visible structural rules" (Day, 1990, p. 113). These modern materials are also often used in a deceptive way–vinyl siding replicating wood–which tends to corrupt the nature of materials. As a result, authenticity is questionable and modern materials tend to "look as fake and hollow as they sound when you tap them" (Day, 1990, p. 116).

Frank Lloyd Wright (1954) stressed the importance of authenticity when he stated that materials should be used "for their own sake." According to Wright, "a stone building will no more be nor will it look like a steel building. A pottery, or terra cotta building, will not be nor should it be like a stone building" (p. 52). Nature had taught him to see "brick as brick." He "learned to see wood as wood . . . for itself" (p. 21). Similarly, the Florida village of Seaside, in its architectural codes, limits the use of materials to those in use before 1940 "to keep the buildings honest" (Mohney, 1991, p. 64). At that time, "materials were what they were" (p. 64). In order to adhere to authenticity, Wright never painted wood, covered it or twisted it out of shape. He often smoothed or stained it, but that was to highlight its natural grain (Twombly, 1979). Nonetheless, Wright did state that even synthetic materials could be used "naturally" if they were used properly and adhered to their defining qualities. This, of course, defies the definition of "naturalness" which is used here. In contrast, Frewald (1989) indicated that natural building materials such as field-stone and wood, as opposed to synthetic materials or those which appear manufactured, enhance preference largely because they serve as connections to the natural environment.

CONCLUDING REMARKS

In sum, a framework for examining homeyness in relation to the exterior of assisted living housing for the elderly is proposed in light of McCracken's (1989) work and other literature that has addressed the meaning of home for the elderly. Specifically, the proposed framework incorporates three overarching themes, including "supportive protection," "human scale," and "naturalness." Previous research has shown that these themes are pertinent to the symbolic nature of homeyness in the context of the single family house, and a few researchers have begun to investigate aspects of these themes in relation to assisted living housing for the elderly.

Gaining a greater understanding of homeyness in relation to assisted living is an important concern. Unlike the nursing home, which is grounded in the medical model and consequently looks and functions like a hospital, assisted living has been promoted as a residential model that blends personal and health care services in a homelike setting. A number of researchers have discussed the importance of a noninstitutional image as one way to create a homelike ambiance (Moore, 1999; Marsden, 1999; Marsden and Kaplan, 1999; Regnier, 1994; Regnier et al., 1995). Such residential references not only impact marketability, they can also affect "attitudes and therefore behaviors of residents, staff, and visitors alike" (Moore, 1999, p. 10). In other words, a place that looks like home may help to set the stage, through symbolic messages, for the operational patterns and activities that must occur for an assisted living residence to function like home as well.

REFERENCES

Alexander, C., Ishikawa, S. and Silverstein, M., with Jacobsen, M., Fiskdahl-King, I. and Angel, Shlomo. (1977). *A pattern language.* New York: Oxford University Press.

Altman, I. and Werner, C. M. (Eds.). (1985). *Home environments.* New York: Plenum Press.

American Association of Retired Persons (AARP). (1996). *Understanding senior housing into the next century: Survey of consumer preferences, concerns, and needs.* Washington DC: AARP.

Bloomer, K. C. and Moore, C. W. (1977). *Body, memory, and architecture.* New Haven, CT: Yale University Press.

Boschetti, M. A. (1984). *The older person's emotional attachment to the physical environment of the residential setting.* Doctoral dissertation. The University of Michigan, Ann Arbor, MI.

Brawley, E. (1997). *Designing for Alzheimer's Disease: Strategies for creating better care environments.* New York: John Wiley & Sons, Inc.

Brummett, W. (1997). *The essence of home: Design solutions for assisted living housing.* New York: Van Nostrand Reinhold.

Calkins, M. P. (1988). *Designing for dementia: Planning environments for the elderly and confused.* Owings Mills: National Health Publishing.

Cherulnik, P. D. and Wilderman, S. K. (1986). Symbols of status in urban neighborhoods: Contemporary perceptions of nineteenth-century Boston. *Environment and Behavior, 18,* 604-622.

Clark, C. E. (1986). *The American family home.* Chapel Hill, NC: University of North Carolina Press.

Cohen, U. and Weisman, G. D. (1991). *Holding on to home: Designing environments for people with dementia.* Baltimore, MD: The Johns Hopkins University Press.

Cooper, C. (1974). The house as symbol of self. In J. D. Lang, C. Burnette, W. Moleski and D. Vachon (Eds.), *Designing for human behavior: Architecture and the behavioral sciences* (pp. 130-146). Stroudsburg, PA: Dowden, Hutchinson & Ross, Inc.

Day, C. (1993). *Places of the soul: Architecture and environmental design as a healing art.* London: Thorsons.

Despres, C. (1991). The meaning of home: Literature review and directions for future research and theoretical development. *The Journal of Architectural and Planning Research,* 8 (2), 96-114.

Devlin, A. S. (1994). Children's housing preferences: Regional, socioeconomic, and adult comparison. *Environment and Behavior,* 26 (4), 527-559.

Dovey, K. (1985). Home and homelessness. In I. Altman and C. M. Werner (Eds.), *Home environments* (pp. 33-64). New York: Plenum Press.

Duncan, J., Jr. (1973). Landscape taste as a symbol of group identity: A Westchester County Village. *The Geographical Review,* 63, 334-355.

Dupuis A. and Thorns, D. C. (1996). Meaning of *home* for older *home* owners. *Housing Studies,* 11, 485-501.

Fogel, B. S. (1992, Spring). Psychological aspects of staying at home. *Generations,* pp. 15-19.

Frewald, D. B. (1989). *Preferences for older buildings: A psychological approach to architectural design.* Doctoral Dissertation. The University of Michigan, Ann Arbor, MI.

Fusch, R. and Ford, L. (1986). Architecture and the geography of the American City. *The Geographical Review,* 79, 324-340.

Hoglund, J. D. and Ledewitz, S. D. (1999). Designing to meet the needs of people with Alzheimer's Disease. In B. Schwarz and R. Brent (Eds.), *Aging, autonomy, and architecture: Advances in assisted living* (pp. 229-261). Baltimore, MD: The Johns Hopkins University Press.

Howell, S. (1985). Home: A source of meaning in elders' lives. *Generations,* 9 (3), 58-60.

Kaplan, S. and Kaplan, R. (1978). *Humanscape: Environments for People.* (Republished, Ann Arbor, MI: Ulrich's, 1982).

Kaplan, S. and Kaplan, R. (1982). *Cognition and Environment: Functioning in an Uncertain World.* New York: Praeger. (Republished by Ulrich's: Ann Arbor, MI).

Kaplan, S., Kaplan, R. and Wendt, J. S. (1972). Rated preferences and complexity for natural and urban visual material. *Perception and Psychophysics,* 12, 354-356.

Kavanaugh, G. (1983). Foreword. In C. W. Moore, K. Smith, and P. Becker (Eds.), *Home Sweet Home* (pp. 11-13). New York: Rizzoli International Publications, Inc.

Kemp, J. (1987). *American vernacular: Regional influences in architecture and interior design.* New York: Viking Penguin, Inc.

Kron, J. (1990). Real living: An anthropologist uncovers what some decorators see as a dark side: Homeyness. *The New York Times,* p. D1.

Küller, R. (1988). Environmental activation of old persons suffering from senile dementia. In H. van Hoogdalem, N. L. Prak, R. J. M. van der Voordt and H. B. R. van Wegen (Eds.), *Looking back to the future,* Proceeding of the Tenth Biennial Conference of the International Association for the Study of People and Their Physical Surroundings, (133-139). Delft, The Netherlands: Delft University Press.

Lang, J. (1987). *Creating architectural theory: The role of the behavioral sciences in environmental design.* New York: Van Nostrand Reinhold Company.

Langdon, P. (1982, April 22). Suburbanites pick favorite home styles. *The New York Times,* p. C12.

Lansing, J. B., Marans, R. W. and Zehner, R. B. (1970). *Planned residential environments*. Ann Arbor, MI: The Survey Research Center, University of Michigan.

Marsden, J. P. (1999). Older persons' and family members' perceptions of assisted living. *Environment and Behavior*, 31 (1), 84-106.

Marsden, J. P. and Kaplan, R. (1999). Communicating homeyness from the outside: Elderly people's perceptions of assisted living. In B. Schwarz and R. Brent (Eds.), *Aging, autonomy, and architecture: Advances in assisted living* (pp. 207-228). Baltimore, MD: The Johns Hopkins University Press.

Materiality and Resistance. (1994, May). *The Architectural Review*, 194, pp. 4-5.

McCracken, G. (1989). Homeyness: A cultural account of the constellation of consumer goods and meanings. In E. Hirschman (Ed.), *Interpretive consumer culture*. Provo, UT: Association for Consumer Research.

Mohney, D. (1991). Interview with Andres Duany. In D. Mohney and K. Easterling (Eds.), *Seaside* (pp. 62-73). Princeton, NJ: Princeton Architectural Press.

Moore, C. and Allen, G. (1976). *Dimensions: Space, shape & scale in architecture*. New York: Architectural Record Books.

Moore, C., Allen, G. and Lyndon, D. (1974). *The place of houses*. New York: Holt, Rinehart and Winston.

Moore, J. (2000). Placing *home* in context. *Journal of Environmental Psychology*, 20, 207-217.

Moore, K. D. (1999). *Towards a language of assisted living: Understanding the physical setting through benchmarking*. Milwaukee, WI: Institute on Aging and Environment, University of Wisconsin-Milwaukee.

Morgan, J. (1996). *If these walls had ears: The biography of a house*. New York: Warner Books, Inc.

Mugerauer, R. (1993). Toward an architectural vocabulary: The porch as a between. In D. Seamon (Ed.), *Dwelling, seeing, and designing: Toward a phenomenological ecology* (pp. 103-128). New York: State University of New York Press.

Nasar, J. L. (1993). Connotative meanings of house styles. In E. G. Arias (Ed.), *The meaning and use of housing* (pp. 143-167). Brookfield, VT: Ashgate Publishing Company.

Nassauer, J. I. (1995). Messy ecosystem, orderly frames. *Landscape Journal*, 161-170.

Norris-Baker, C. and Scheidt, R. J. (1994). From "our town" to "ghost town"?: The changing context of home for rural elders. *Journal of International Aging and Human Development*, 38 (3), 181-202.

O'Bryant, S. L. (1983). The subjective value of "home" to older homeowners. *Journal of Housing for the Elderly*, 1 (1), 29-43.

Orr, F. (1985). *Scale in architecture*. New York: Van Nostrand Reinhold Company.

Pastalan, L. A. and Schwarz, B. (1993). The meaning of home in ecogenic housing: A new concept for elderly women. In H. C. Dandekar (Ed.), *Shelter, women and development*, (pp. 402-407). Ann Arbor, MI: Wahr Publishing.

Purcell, A. T. and Nasar, J. L. (1992). Experiencing other people's houses: A model of similarities and differences in environmental experience. *Journal of Environmental Psychology*, 12, 199-211.

Rapoport, A. (1985). Thinking about home environments: A conceptual framework. In I. Altman and C. M. Werner (Eds.), *Home environments* (pp. 255-286). New York: Plenum Press.

Rapoport, A. (1969). *House, form and culture*. Englewood Cliffs, NJ: Prentice-Hall, Inc.

Regnier, V. (1999). The definition and evolution of assisted living within a changing system of long-term care. In B. Schwarz and R. Brent (Eds.) *Aging, autonomy, and architecture: Advances in assisted living* (pp. 229-261). Baltimore, MD: The Johns Hopkins University Press

Regnier, V. (1994). *Assisted living housing for the elderly: Design innovations from the United States and Europe.* New York: Van Nostrand Rinehold.

Regnier, V., Hamilton, J. & Yatabe, S. (1995). *Assisted living for the frail: Innovations in design, management, and financing.* New York: Columbia University Press.

Robinson, J. (1989). Architecture as a medium for culture: Public institution and private house. In S. M. Low and E. Chambers (Eds.), *Housing, culture, and design* (pp. 253-279). Philadelphia, PA: University of Pennsylvania Press.

Rowles, G. D. (1983). Place and personal identity in old age: Observations from Appalachia. *Journal of Environmental Psychology, 3,* 299-313.

Rowles, G. D. (1987). A place to call home. In L. L. Carstensen and B. A. Edelstein (Eds.), *Handbook of clinical gerontology* (pp. 335-353). New York: Pergamon Press.

Royse, D. C. (1969). *Social inferences via environmental cues.* Doctoral dissertation, MIT, Cambridge, MA.

Rubinstein R. L. (1989). The home environments of older people: A description of the psychosocial process linking person to place. *Journal of Gerontology, 44* (2), 545-553.

Sadalla, E. K. and Sheets, V. L. (1993). Symbolism in building materials: Self-presentational and cognitive components. *Environment and Behavior, 25* (2), 155-180.

Sadalla, E. K., Vershure, B. and Burroughs, J. (1987). Identity symbolism in housing. *Environment and Behavior, 19* (5), 569-587.

Saegert, S. (1985). The role of housing in the experience of dwelling. In I. Altman and C. M. Werner (Eds.), *Home environments* (pp. 287-309). New York: Plenum Press.

Schwarz, B. (1999). Assisted living: An evolving place type. In B. Schwarz and R. Brent (Eds.). *Aging, autonomy, and architecture: Advances in assisted living* (pp. 185-206). Baltimore, MD: The Johns Hopkins University Press.

Sixsmith, A. J. and Sixsmith, J. A. (1991). Transitions in home experience in later life. *The Journal of Architectural and Planning Research, 8* (3), 181-191.

Tognoli, J. (1987). Residential environments. In D. Stokols and I. Altman (Eds), *Handbook of environmental psychology* (pp. 655-690). New York: John Wiley & Sons, Inc.

Twombly, R. C. (1979). *Frank Lloyd Wright: His life and his architecture.* New York: John Wiley & Sons.

United States Conference of Mayors (USCM) and United States Department of Housing and Urban Development (HUD) (1977). *Developing a local housing strategy: A guidebook for local government.*

van Vliet, W. (1998). Home. In W. van Vliet (Ed.), *The encyclopedia of housing* (pp. 222-223). Thousand Oaks, CA: SAGE Publications, Inc.

Werthman, C. S. (1969). *The social meaning of the physical environment.* Ann Arbor, MI: University Microfilms, Inc.

Wilson, K. (1995). Assisted living as a model of care delivery. In L. Gamroth, J. Semradek, and E. Tornquist (Eds.), *Enhancing autonomy in long-term care: Concepts and strategies.* New York: Springer.

Wright, F. L. (1954). *The natural house.* New York: Horizon Press, Inc.

Zeisel, J. (1999). Life-quality Alzheimer care in assisted living. In B. Schwarz and R. Brent (Eds.), *Aging, autonomy, and architecture: Advances in assisted living* (pp. 110-129). Baltimore, MD: The Johns Hopkins University Press.

Chapter 7

Linking Housing and Services for Low-Income Elderly: Lessons from 1994 Best Practice Award Winners

Beth Madvin Cox

SUMMARY. This research was designed to identify characteristics of the Department of Housing and Urban Development's (HUD) Best Practice Award winners. Lessons learned from award winners can be used to improve methods of linking housing and community services for low-income elders. Data were derived from applications for the HUD 1994 Best Practice Award competition. Characteristics that differentiated award winners from non-winners were identified. Findings suggested that award winners provided access to a significantly greater number of supportive and health services. Findings also suggest that award winners were more adept at utilizing community resources. The results of this

---

At the time of this writing, Beth Madvin Cox, PhD, was a Post Doctoral Fellow in the School of Nursing at Oregon Health Sciences University, Portland, Oregon.

This article is adapted from a dissertation conducted at the University of Southern California.

The writing of this manuscript was supported by National Institutes of Health, National Research Award T32 NR07048, from the Oregon Health Sciences University.

[Haworth co-indexing entry note]: "Chapter 7. Linking Housing and Services for Low-Income Elderly: Lessons from 1994 Best Practice Award Winners." Cox, Beth Madvin. Co-published simultaneously in *Journal of Housing for the Elderly* (The Haworth Press, Inc.) Vol. 15. No. 1/2. 2001. pp. 97-110; and: *Assisted Living: Sobering Realities* (ed: Benyamin Schwarz) The Haworth Press, Inc., 2001. pp. 97-110. Single or multiple copies of this article are available for a fee from The Haworth Document Delivery Service [1-800-342-9678, 9:00 a.m. - 5:00 p.m. (EST). E-mail address: getinfo@haworthpressinc.com].

97

study are useful in the continued development of comprehensive aging-in-place programs for low-income elderly. *[Article copies available for a fee from The Haworth Document Delivery Service: 1-800-342-9678. E-mail address: <getinfo@haworthpressinc.com> Website: <http://www. HaworthPress.com>* © *2001 by The Haworth Press, Inc. All rights reserved.]*

KEYWORDS. Supportive housing, elderly, community-based services, aging-in-place

INTRODUCTION

The need for development of long-term care options for low-income elders is an issue of increasing concern. The proportion of elderly persons in the United States' population is growing. By 2030 those over 65 will represent about 20% of the population, and by the year 2050 it is projected that individuals over 85 will represent about 5 percent of the total population (U.S. Bureau of the Census, 1996). With the increase in sheer numbers of elderly comes a rise in the number of individuals needing assistance with activities of daily living (ADLs) (Whittle and Goldenberg, 1996). This will result in an increase in the already existing need for enhanced long-term care service options.

In recent years the types of settings for providing long-term care have proliferated, and a continuum of long-term care has developed. On one end of the spectrum, pressures to reduce hospital lengths of stay have resulted in the emergence of special care units in nursing homes, as well as in-home treatments of chronic conditions that have traditionally been provided in the hospital. On the other end of the spectrum, added to traditional nursing home and home care settings, are "demedicalized" community-based, long-term care environments (Binstock & Spector, 1997). The supportive services offered in these settings vary considerably in physical design, level of services provided, populations served, and overall quality of care (Pynoos and Golant, 1996). Community-based demedicalized settings offering supportive services include assisted living complexes, continuing care retirement communities, board and care homes, and supportive housing.

The proportion of persons aged 65 and older having a pre-tax income of less than 200 percent of the poverty threshold is 38 percent (Binstock & Spector, 1997). Because cost of long-term care is high and rising fast (Binstock & Spector, 1997), many long-term care options are accessible only to those who can afford the expense (Pynoos, 1994). The cost of most long-term care options means that some low-income elders continue to live independently beyond their ability to care for themselves, while others enter nursing homes but do not require the level of care provided in that setting (Struyk, Page, Newman, Carroll, Makiko, Cohen, & Wright, 1989).

SUPPORTIVE HOUSING

Supportive housing is a long-term care option for individuals who are not in need of intensive or extensive medical care and who are able to function independently with some support. This housing option, which provides access to health and social services, can enable elders to remain in their residence of choice while receiving necessary services, maximizing their own efforts to retain functional independence (Heumann & Boldy, 1993). Multi-unit housing with supportive services is available through private, non-profit, and public sponsors including the Department of Housing and Urban Development (HUD). The research study described in this article focuses on the identification of characteristics of HUD subsidized multi-unit housing which provide elderly residents with access to an array of supportive services. It is hoped that the identification of these characteristics will enhance the future development of multi-unit housing with linkages to supportive services.

Supportive housing can be planned and built with the intent to provide services, or preexisting facilities originally developed for an independent population can have services added as residents age. Facility management or sponsors can develop supportive programs through a variety of different methods: providing the services directly, relying extensively on outside community resources, or employing a mix of the two. In federally subsidized housing facilities, supportive services are often provided by charitable organizations as well as state and local agencies, such as Area Agencies on Aging.

Linking housing with community-based health and social services is a means of providing access to the support needed for low-income elders who desire to age-in-place. Supportive housing has the potential to delay moves to higher levels of care, such as nursing homes; to fulfill the strong preference people have to remain in their own homes (Pynoos & Golant, 1996); to enhance quality of life (Kemper, Applebaum, & Harrington, 1987); and to increase satisfaction with life (Hughes, Conrad, Manheim, & Edelmann, 1988; Kemper et al., 1987; Weissert, Cready, & Pawelek, 1988). There is also evidence to suggest that supportive housing can help prolong independence, reduce isolation, and increase opportunities for socialization among residents (Kaye, Monk, & Diamond, 1985).

There are different levels of support services provided in supportive housing. Some housing facilities may provide access to a minimal number of services while others may provide a wide range. For the purposes of this research, a basic level of supportive housing is defined as independent apartment living supplemented by non-medical services, including housekeeping, transportation, at least one meal daily, and some level of personal care (Nachison, 1995). A comprehensive level of supportive housing involves access to the provision of an increased variety of on-site services, including physical and mental health programs, emergency response systems, an on-site beautician, or a convenience store (Miller, 1991).

On-site health services can greatly benefit elders who wish to maintain independent living. Access to health services can positively influence physical and mental health because the early identification of health and service needs can result in interventions that prolong physical independence and enhance an elder's ability to remain independent. A brief geriatric screening assessment can detect unrecognized and treatable problems, even among relatively healthy older adults (Fabacher, Josephson, Pietruszka, Linderborn, Morely, & Rubenstein, 1994). Visiting health professionals can identify elders with early functional problems and assist in targeting strategies to prevent progression of disability and improve the individual's function (Fried & Guralnik, 1997). Higher levels of functioning are associated with higher levels of life-satisfaction and emotional well-being (Whittle & Goldenberg, 1996).

Supportive housing is attractive from a policy perspective. Potential for cost savings exists with supportive housing because it promotes independent living, eliminates the need for expensive on-site nursing care, and brings in professional support only at the level required to meet the need of the individual (Heumann, 1991). Although Weissert et al. (1988) argue that there is little evidence that subsidized home care reduces aggregate long-term care costs, the work of Greene et al. suggests that if home care services were more tightly targeted to appropriate individuals, the potential for program level cost savings might be significantly improved (Greene, Lovely, Miller, & Ondrich, 1995; Greene, Lovely, Ondrich, & Laditka, 1998). Thus, supportive housing programs should target elders who can live independently with some support.

Supportive housing is a cost-effective alternative to higher levels of care for a select population which includes elders at risk for placement in facilities providing higher levels of care, such as institutionalization, but who are not in need of extensive or intensive medical care. Cost savings would accrue if those who otherwise would be placed in nursing homes could be successfully targeted and placed in a non-institutional environment (Heumann, 1991).

The increasing population of low-income elders renders critical the need to organize creative means in the development of supportive service provision. A question arises as to the best way to provide supportive housing to low-income elders in housing originally designed for independent residents. A first step would be to examine existing successful models. Winners of the 1994 HUD Best Practice award provide excellent models to examine in the pursuit of ideas for the enhanced development of low-cost programs for low-income elders. This article analyzes supportive service provision in HUD subsidized housing. Practices of award winning facilities will be identified in order to facilitate replication in other settings.

HUD 1994 BEST PRACTICE AWARD

In 1994, HUD and the Administration on Aging (AoA) conducted a Best Practice Award competition in order to recognize and award HUD subsidized multi-unit housing facilities that offered supportive service programs to elderly residents. The search for nominees was publicized nationwide. To be eligible for nomination the facility must have been HUD subsidized and designated or approved as housing for elders and disabled. A total of 120 facilities were nominated or self-nominated for the HUD Best Practice Award. In 1995, the winners of the HUD competition were picked after panels of experts from HUD and AoA established selection criteria and met to review and rank applications. These criteria included:

- Facility provides or makes available, directly or through third parties, a core service package (one or more meals per day, access to housekeeping and personal assistance).
- Facility provides a wide range of accessible, affordable, and adaptable services in addition to the core.
- Facility demonstrates coordinated efforts that are working well, emphasizing cooperative efforts between the housing provider and community agencies.

Twenty-three winners were selected by the judges. Each of the 23 winning facilities were ascertained to have established effective approaches to comprehensive service provision, providing a wide range of health and social services, and demonstrating success in linking low-income elders with community-based services.

HYPOTHESES

The purpose of the research reported here was to ascertain whether there were statistical differences between HUD Best Practice award winners and non-winners, and to identify salient characteristics of winners. It is expected that lessons learned from the identification of characteristics of winners will enhance future development of supportive housing for low-income elders.

Two hypotheses directed this research. Hypotheses were based on the assumption that winners of the HUD Best Practice award provided more services and better utilized community resources in order to do so.

Hypothesis One: Winners of the HUD best practice award offer a greater number of supportive, clinical, and ancillary services to residents than non-winners.

Hypothesis Two: Winners better utilize community resources. Winners will be more apt to use outside providers in the delivery of services than non-winners and will use more providers in the provision of individual services than non-winners.

METHODS

Sample

Of the 120 HUD Best Practice Award nominees, 117 were included in the sample. One facility was excluded because it housed developmentally disabled non-elderly. Two facilities were excluded because they were missing information considered vital to this study. In the research study that follows, award winners (n = 23) are compared to non-winners (n = 94).

The application process for the HUD Best Practice award required each nominee to submit a narrative describing services offered and mechanisms for the provision of each service. Discrete and continuous variables used in this research study were identified and classified based on information provided on each application form.

For purposes of analysis, services provided were divided into three categories: supportive services, health services, and ancillary services (Figure 1). All services listed in Figure 1 emerged after analysis of every application packet. Every service listed was provided by at least one nominee. Supportive services are described in the column headed "supportive services." "Health services," described in the second column, are defined as on-site health related services delivered by visiting nurses, physicians, or other health professionals. "Ancillary services," described in the third column, do not specifically address deficiencies in activities of daily living or health needs; however, their provision further enables the individual to satisfy social and other needs on the premises.

Variables consisted of data pertaining to: whether particular service was provided, how many services were provided; who provided each service (sponsor or outside provider), and how many providers were involved in the provision of each service (single, multiple). For each nominee the services offered in each category (Figure 1) were counted. Each application was examined to identify whether, and how, each of the services in Figure 1 was provided. A service was considered "provided" when the housing facility offered access to the service, regardless of the role of the facility in the provision of the service. A nominee's winner/non-winner status was coded as well.

Descriptive and non-parametric statistics were used to analyze data comparing winners to non-winners because the sample was not drawn using random sampling methods. The level of significance was set at the .05 level for all statistical tests. Wilcoxon Mann-Whitney and crosstabs were performed to test

FIGURE 1. Three Categories of Possible Services

Supportive Services	Health Services	Ancillary Services
• Service Coordination	• Evaluations & Referral	• Recreational & Educational
• Housekeeping Services	• Vital Sign Checks	• Tenants Association
• Home Health Services	• Glucose Checks	• Financial Counseling
• Personal Care	• Nutritional Counseling	• Legal Assistance
• Home Delivered Meals	• Flu Shots/Clinic	• Beautician
• Congregate Meals	• Vision Checks	• Library
• Security Services	• Hearing Screenings	• Banking Services
• Transportation	• Podiatry	• Convenience Store
• Mental Health Services	• Medication Monitoring	• Senior Companion
• Adult Day Care	• Dental	
• On-site visiting		
Physician		
Nurse		
Podiatrist		
Optometrist		

the null hypothesis that there was no difference between winners and non-winners.

Limitations of the data set may have affected results somewhat. First, facilities may have referred to the same services by different names or may have referred to different services by the same name: data in this analysis were coded as stated on the application forms. Second, specific services may have been listed twice under different service categories (see Figure 1). For example, a visiting optometrist was counted as a supportive service while vision checks were counted as a health service.

FINDINGS

Winners Provide More Services

The first hypothesis was supported. Winners of the 1994 HUD Best Practice award provided access to a greater number of supportive, clinical, and ancillary services (Figure 2). Winners provided linkages to a greater number of supportive services ($p < .01$), and were more likely to provide on-site nursing services (p < .01), mental health services (p < .05), and security services (p < .05) (Figure 3a). Winners offered a greater number of health services than non-winners (p < .01), were more likely to provide health services in general (p < .05), and were more inclined to provide vital sign checks (p < .01), nurse assessment and referral (p < .01), podiatry (p < .05), and nutritional counseling (p < .05). Further, thirty percent of winners provided a designated on-site clinic space for visiting health professionals, versus seven percent of non-winners (p < .01) (Figure 3b).

Winners offered a greater number of ancillary services than non-winners (p < .05), and are significantly more likely to provide an on-site beautician (p < .05), on-site convenience store (p < .05), and financial counseling (p < .05). Moreover, winners were significantly more likely (39%) than non-winners (7%) to be located adjacent to a senior center, area agency on aging, or other resource center (p < .01) (Figure 3c).

WINNERS BETTER UTILIZE COMMUNITY RESOURCES

The second hypothesis was based on the assumption that winners would better utilize community resources, using more outside providers and multiple providers in the provision of each service when compared to non-winners. This hypothesis was supported. Winners more often used outside providers (Figure 4) and multiple providers (Figure 5) in service provision. Winners

FIGURE 2. Mean Number of Services Provided

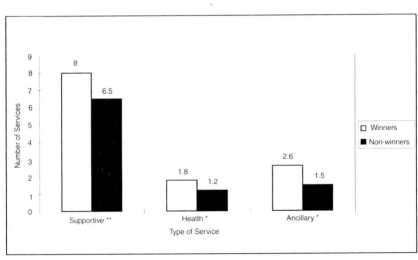

* p < .05   ** p < .01

FIGURE 3a. Winners Provide More Supportive Services

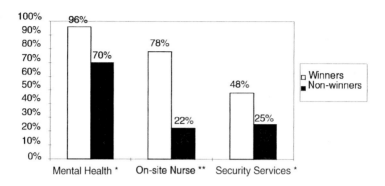

FIGURE 3b. Winners Provide More Health Services

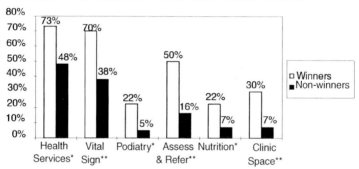

FIGURE 3c. Winners Provide More Ancillary Services

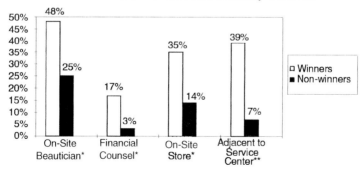

FIGURE 4. Use of Outside Providers

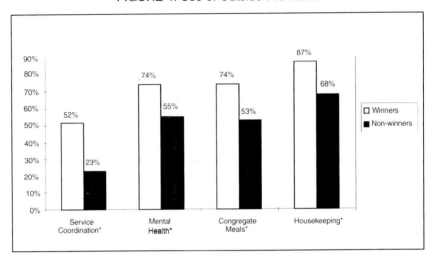

* p < .05 ** p < .01
May not add up to 100% due to lack of responses

FIGURE 5. Use of Multiple Service Providers

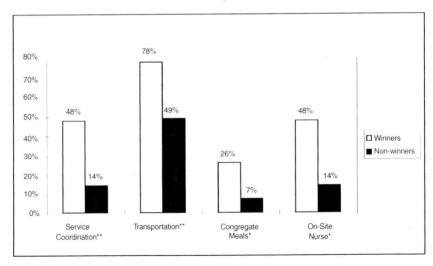

* p < .05 ** p < .01
May not add up to 100% due to lack of responses

used outside providers more often in the provision: of service coordination (p < .05), congregate meals (p < .05) housekeeping (p < .05) and mental health services (p < .05). Winners were more likely to utilize multiple providers in the provision of: service coordination (p < .01), transportation (p < .01), congregate meals (p < .05), and on-site nurse (p < .05).

DISCUSSION

Findings of this research demonstrated that HUD Best Practice award winners provided access to a significantly greater number of supportive, clinical, and ancillary services, and were more adept at managing community resources, utilizing more outside and multiple providers.

It cannot be assumed that it is the proclivity of the facility management that leads to greater success in service provision. Before we seek to develop innovative methods in the development of supportive housing, we must first understand the circumstances that render one multi-unit housing facility more successful than another. For example, is it the facility staff or the community service agency taking the lead in organizing service provision?

Winners were significantly more likely than non-winners to be located adjacent to community centers. This geographical advantage may explain the success of some facilities but does not explain the success of the majority of winners that are not adjacent to a senior or community center. Perhaps winners who were not adjacent to resource centers better planned, coordinated, and utilized community resources; these actions may have led to the ability to provide a greater number of health and social services. Or, winning facilities may have had more on-site space available for clinic and other service programs. Future research should examine whether better planning and resource utilization on the part of housing management, better service delivery techniques on the part of a proactive provider, or a combination of these two processes are responsible for the provision of a greater range of long-term care services.

Winners used more multiple and outside providers in the provision of services. This may demonstrate a greater ability to coordinate outside resources. However, the difference in who was reported by nominees as having provided specific services may be due more to environmental circumstances surrounding the facility rather than better community resource utilization. What appears to be better utilization of outside and multiple providers by winners may instead point to greater availability of community resources and outside providers. Non-winners may use their own staff to provide services, and may provide fewer services because they are not near service centers or other available resources. A limitation to the database used in this analysis was that it was not possible to test whether characteristics of the community, or characteristics of the services available within that community, contributed to the ease or difficulty of accessing services. A given community may be more charitable, more resourceful, more economically advantaged, or may harbor greater commitment to the elderly. These are all possibilities that may be evaluated in future studies.

DEVELOPING SUPPORTIVE HOUSING
FOR LOW-INCOME ELDERS

It is possible to provide access to a full range of long-term care support services to low-income elders in multi-unit housing. Existing community resources can be linked with multi-unit housing, enabling elders to function as independently as possible in their own residences. Housing sponsors and managers should understand that they can create a supportive environment for aging residents by making use of services offered through local public and non-profit service agencies. But why should housing sponsors or managers bring supportive services in housing intended for the independent resident? What are advantages to housing providers? First, integrating supportive services into the facility, such as health and homemaker services, can reduce the incidence of resident turnover and improve overall apartment maintenance. At the same time, a facility that offers services to its residents will increase its marketability in the local housing market. Perhaps the greatest advantage of all lies with the simple fact that supportive services will enhance a resident's quality of life by fostering independence and enabling them to age-in-place (American Association of Homes for the Aging, 1993).

For an existing facility designed with an independent population in mind, start-up and operational costs, management time and energy, and increased exposure may make direct service provision difficult. A housing facility which was not purposely designed to house and support frail elders may find it more advantageous to assist in linking residents with community-based services rather than attempting to provide services from within (American Association of Homes for the Aging, 1993).

In order to begin establishment of linkages with community based providers, housing sponsors can contact local agencies, such as Adult and Family Services or Area Agencies on Aging. Also, to support linkages between the housing facility and community service providers, the sponsor or management can offer use of space to home health agencies, senior centers, adult day care, and others (American Association of Homes for the Aging, 1993). Facilities without extra or common space can address this issue by converting existing units into clinic or common space, or by adding on to the facility.

Low-income elders have few housing options when in need of supportive services. Innovative strategies that link housing and services are necessary to enable this population to age in their own residences. The identification of characteristics of winners of the 1994 HUD Best Practice Award provides insight into program development for the low-income population. Winners better utilized existing resources by using more multiple and outside providers and provided more supportive, health, and ancillary services. Other multi-unit housing facilities can emulate Best Practice Award winners by assisting elderly residents in linking with available community-based services.

In this era of aging demographics and dwindling public resources, strategies for future housing and long-term care innovations must be developed. New options must be developed, not only in the attempt to decrease societal costs, but also to provide options to elders who may benefit psychologically and functionally from programs that encourage aging in place. Success in this arena is dependent upon both research and practice as gerontologists and policy makers seek new methods of utilizing existing resources.

REFERENCES

American Association of Homes for the Aging (1993). *Critical Link: Building Supportive Environments for Low-Income Elderly.*

Binstock, R., and Spector, W. (1997). Five Priority Areas for Research on Long-Term Care. *Health Services Research* 32: 5.

Fabacher, D., Josephson, K., Pietruszka, F., Linderborn, K., Morely, J., & Rubenstein, L. (1994). An in-home preventative assessment program for independent older adults: A randomized controlled trial. *Journal of American Geriatrics Society,* 42 (6): 630-638.

Fried, L., & Guralnik, J. (1997). Disability in older adults: Evidence regarding significance, etiology, and risk. *Journal American Geriatrics Society,* 45, 92-100.

Greene, V., Lovely, M., Miller, M., & Ondrich, J. (1995). Reducing nursing home use through community long-term care: An optimization analysis. *Journals of Gerontology,* 50B (40), S259-268.

Greene, V., Lovely, M., Ondrich, J., & Laditka, S. (1998). Can home care services achieve cost savings in long term care for older people. *Journals of Gerontology,* 51B (4), S228-238.

Heumann, L. F. (1991). A cost comparison of congregate housing and long-term care facilities for elderly residents with comparable support needs in 1985 and 1990. *Journal of Housing for the Elderly,* 9 (1/2).

Heumann L., & Boldy, D. (1993). *Aging in Place with Dignity.* Praeger Publishers, CT.

Hughes, S. L., Conrad, K. L., Manheim, L. M., & Edelman, P. L. (1988). Impact of long-term home care on mortality, functional status, and unmet needs, *Health Services Research,* 23, 269-294.

Kaye, L.W., Monk, A., & Diamond, B.E. (1985). *The enrichment of residential housing stock for elderly tenants: A national analysis and case feasibility study.* New York, Columbia University Press.

Kemper, P., Applebaum, R., & Harrington, M. (1987). Community care demonstrations: What have we learned? *Health Care Financing Review,* 8 (4).

Miller, J. (1991). *Community based long-term care.* Sage Publications.

Nachison, Jerold. (1995). Who pays: The congregate housing question. *Generations,* Spring, p. 34.

Pynoos, J. (1994). Housing Policy for the elderly. In P. Kim (Ed.), *Services to the aging and aged: Public policies and programs.* New York, NY: Garland Publishing.

Pynoos, J. (1992). Linking federally assisted housing with services for frail older people. *Journal of Aging & Social Policy,* 4 (3 & 4), 157-177.

Pynoos, J., & Golant, S. (1996). Housing and living arrangements for the elderly. In R. Binstock, J. Schulz, & L. George (Eds.), *Handbook of Aging and the Social Sciences.* Academic Press, Inc.

Struyk, R.J., Page, D.B., Newman, S., Carroll, M., Makiko, V., Cohen, B., & Wright, P. (1989). *Providing supportive services to the frail elderly in federally assisted housing.* Urban Institute Press.

U.S. Bureau of the Census *Current Population Reports, Special Studies, P23-190, 65+ in the United States.* U.S. Government Printing Office, Washington, DC.

Weissert, W. G., Cready, C. M., and Pawelek, E. (1988). The past and future of home and community based long-term care. *Milbank Memorial Fund Quarterly,* 66, 309-388.

Whittle, H., & Goldenberg, D. (1996). Functional health status and instrumental activities of daily living performance in non-institutionalized elderly people. *Journal of Advanced Nursing,* 23, 220-227.

Chapter 8

Exploring the Housing Assistance Needs of Elderly Renters

Amy S. Bogdon
Harold Katsura
Maris Mikelsons

SUMMARY. The economic well-being of the elderly population has risen dramatically in recent decades, yet the elderly are more likely to be poor or near poor than are most other adult age groups. The review of evidence on different measures of poverty and housing problems shows that significant segments of the elderly population–in particular, many elderly renters–have unmet needs for housing assistance. The diversity of need among the elderly suggests that elderly housing assistance should be focused on subgroups, which are currently not well served by assistance programs. *[Article copies available for a fee from The Haworth Document Delivery Service: 1-800-342-9678. E-mail address: <getinfo@ haworthpressinc.com> Website: <http://www.HaworthPress.com> © 2001 by The Haworth Press, Inc. All rights reserved.]*

KEYWORDS. Housing policy, entitlement programs, poverty

Amy S. Bogdon is currently Director of Housing Economics Research at the Fannie Mae Foundation. This article is based on research conducted while she was employed by the Urban Institute. Harold Katsura and Maris Mikelsons are Research Associates at The Urban Institute.

[Haworth co-indexing entry note]: "Chapter 8. Exploring the Housing Assistance Needs of Elderly Renters." Bogdon, Amy S., Harold Katsura, and Maris Mikelsons. Co-published simultaneously in *Journal of Housing for the Elderly* (The Haworth Press, Inc.) Vol. 15, No. 1/2, 2001, pp. 111-130; and: *Assisted Living: Sobering Realities* (ed: Benyamin Schwarz) The Haworth Press, Inc., 2001, pp. 111-130. Single or multiple copies of this article are available for a fee from The Haworth Document Delivery Service [1-800-342-9678, 9:00 a.m. - 5:00 p.m. (EST). E-mail address: getinfo@haworthpressinc.com].

INTRODUCTION

The challenge of adequately housing the nation's aging population is growing each day. There are now more elderly persons than ever in the history of the United States. In 1999, there were about 34.5 million people aged 65 and over, constituting about 12.7 percent of the entire population. The Bureau of the Census estimates that this group will grow to almost 40 million people by the year 2010. Increases in the total number of elderly people will be accompanied by increased racial and ethnic diversity among the elderly. In 1990, members of minority groups accounted for 9.8 percent of all elderly. This share is expected to increase to 16.5 percent by the year 2030.

The income and well-being of the elderly in the United States have improved dramatically in the past sixty years. In 1939, nearly four of every five elderly persons were poor compared to only about one in eight by 1984. Although the elderly as a group have improved their economic standing relative to other age groups, some segments of the elderly population experience high rates of poverty and have a high likelihood of living in housing that is unaffordable or physically inadequate.

Policies to assist those facing serious housing problems do not function in the same manner as income assistance programs. Federal rental housing assistance is a rationed program rather than an entitlement given to all households who meet the eligibility criteria.[1] Families (and elderly or handicapped single persons) with incomes below 80 percent of the HUD-adjusted area median are eligible for housing assistance, and until recently, the federal preference system gave priority to those with "worst case" needs.[2]

This assessment of elderly housing assistance needs focuses on the diversity of need within the elderly and other age groups. It begins by comparing several measures of poverty across different age groups. The first section below examines recent poverty rates as measured by the government, looks at the share of people of different ages classified as "very poor" or "near poor," compares household poverty rates and relative incomes by age group, and concludes with a review of the literature on the persistence of poverty among different groups. The next section of the article focuses on the housing problems and housing assistance needs of households of different ages. It compares the share of owners and renters who experience one of three housing problems and the incidence of different housing problems by age. The article concludes with a review of the policy implications of these findings.

POVERTY AND ITS PERSISTENCE AMONG THE ELDERLY

Because poverty studies use a vast number of sometimes conflicting definitions, it is worth taking time at the outset to discuss some technical issues. The official poverty measure is computed by comparing the current money incomes of families with a set of poverty thresholds.[3] If a family's income is below the poverty threshold, all members of the family are classified as poor. The results may be reported in terms of the number of *individuals* or the number of *families* classified as poor.[4] Even when the individual is the unit of analysis, poverty rates may be presented on the basis of family characteristics. For example, some of the tables in this section show the share of *persons* in single parent families who are poor. Since family size varies, this number will not necessarily be the same as the share of single parent *families* who are poor. The choice of a unit of analysis also affects age distributions. In the tables which follow, when individual poverty rates are reported by age, each person is classified according to his or her age. When family or household poverty rates are reported by age, families and households are classified by the age of the head of household, and other family or household members are not counted separately. The elderly account for a larger share of the poor when the family or household, rather than individual, is the unit of analysis because elderly families and households are smaller, on average, than other types of families and households. Although the focus of this article is on renters, much of the existing work on poverty rates considers the total population. The existing work is augmented here by a poverty rate table computed using 1991 American Housing Survey (AHS) data.

Poverty Rates Among Different Groups

The elderly as a group have lower rates of poverty than the total population, but the oldest and youngest age groups are more likely to be poor than those in their middle years. Radner (1992) stresses the importance of examining detailed age groups to obtain a more complete picture of the economic status of the elderly and the non-elderly. He finds great diversity within the elderly population. Married couples have a higher median income than unrelated individuals and the "young old" (age 65 to 74) have a higher median income than those over age 75.

In 1990, the poverty rate for the population over age 65, 12.2 percent, was less than the 13.5 percent poverty rate for the entire population.[5] Poverty rates were lowest for those between the ages of 35 and 59. As Table 1 shows, poverty rates were highest for those under age 18 (20.6 percent), and next highest for those aged 18 to 24 and 75 and over (15.9 and 16.0 percent, respectively). The poverty rates of the elderly may be understated because poverty thresholds are lower for those over age 65.

Poverty rates among the elderly differ by age cohort and household composition. A larger fraction of those over age 75 than those aged 65 to 74 are poor. This is partly due to the fact that successive cohorts among the elderly have experienced improved lifetime economic circumstances. Also, women living alone make up a larger share of those over age 75. They are more likely to be poor than are married couples or men living alone.

TABLE 1. Poverty Rates for Persons by Age in 1990
(Share of Persons Classified as Poor)

By Race and Ethnicity

Age	All Races	White	Black	Hispanic[a]
Under 18	20.6	15.9	44.8	38.4
18 to 24	15.9	13.5	29.6	27.5
25 to 34	12.1	10.0	26.4	23.8
35 to 44	8.5	6.8	19.7	20.6
45 to 54	7.8	6.2	21.1	17.9
55 to 59	9.0	7.4	22.0	18.5
60 to 64	10.3	8.2	27.9	18.1
65 to 74	9.7	7.6	29.6	20.6
75 and over	16.0	13.8	40.6	26.2
Total	13.5	10.7	31.9	28.1
Age 65 and over	12.2	10.1	33.8	22.5

By Race and Gender

Age	All Races	White	Black	Hispanic[a]
Males				
All ages	11.7	9.3	27.9	26.2
Age 65 and over	7.6	5.6	27.8	18.6
65 to 74	6.4	4.5	24.6	18.0
75 and over	9.9	7.8	34.4	20.1
Females				
All ages	15.2	12.0	35.5	29.9
Age 65 and over	15.4	13.2	37.9	25.3
65 to 74	12.3	10.2	33.6	22.7
75 and over	19.5	17.3	43.9	30.1

[a]Persons of Hispanic origin may be of any race.

Source: U.S. Bureau of the Census (1991), income data for 1990 as reported in the March 1991 Current Population Survey.

Elderly poverty rates also vary by race, ethnicity, and gender. In all age groups, blacks and Hispanics have higher poverty rates than whites, and, in most age groups, females have higher poverty rates than males. Among the elderly, these groups also have comparatively higher poverty rates. As the top half of Table 1 illustrates, the overall elderly poverty rate in 1990 was 33.8 percent for blacks and 22.5 percent for Hispanics, compared to 10.1 percent among whites. The bottom half of Table 1 compares poverty rates by race and gender. Only 7.6 percent of elderly males were poor, compared to 15.4 percent of elderly females. Nearly one-fifth of the females over age 75 were poor. Poverty rates for black and Hispanic females were also higher than those for males of the same race or ethnicity.

The elderly are less likely than the total population to be poor or "very poor," but somewhat more likely to be "near poor." About 2.1 percent of the elderly are "very poor," having income below half of the poverty line, compared to 5.2 percent of the total population and 8.8 percent of those under 18 (U.S. Bureau of the Census, 1991). A substantial share of the elderly has income below 150 percent of the poverty line, a classification sometimes referred to as "near poor." Overall, 22.7 percent of the population and 26.3 percent of the elderly are "near poor" by this definition. The diverse circumstances of the elderly are apparent in these data; 34.1 percent of those over age 75 were "near poor" compared to 21.2 percent of those aged 65 to 74. Among those under 18, another age group with low incomes, 34.1 percent were "near poor."

The age pattern of household poverty among renters is similar to the age pattern of poverty among all individuals. Again, poverty rates are highest for the youngest and oldest age groups (Table 2). Nearly one-quarter of renter households and 13.6 percent (not shown) of all households in the 1991 American Housing Survey (AHS) reported incomes below the poverty line.[6] In contrast to the poverty rates computed for individuals, elderly households appear to have slightly higher poverty rates than younger households. Two facts explain this discrepancy: First, among the elderly, single person households are

TABLE 2. Distribution of Income and Poverty Among Renters by Age Group

Age of Head of Renter Household	Household Income Below the Poverty Line	Household Income Below 50% of Adjusted Median	Household Income Above 95% of Adjusted Median
Under 25	37.8%	48.4%	20.9%
25 to 34	21.6	32.6	35.9
35 to 44	20.5	31.4	37.3
45 to 64	22.0	37.4	32.8
65 to 69	21.4	63.5	11.3
70 to 74	25.6	67.7	10.4
75 and older	27.7	74.6	7.4
Under 65	23.8	35.7	33.3
65 and older	25.7	70.3	9.0
All renters	24.0	40.5	30.0

Source: Tabulations of the 1991 AHS by the authors.

more likely to be poor than are married couple households. These individuals account for a larger share of elderly households than of elderly people, raising the elderly household poverty rate. Second, AHS respondents are known to underreport their income, particularly income from sources other than wages or salaries. Since the elderly are more likely to rely on these sources of income than are younger households, underreporting of this type of income will make the elderly appear poorer.

Relative income measures provide another way to compare the well-being of different groups. The third and fourth columns of Table 2 also show part of the income distribution for renter households based on the income eligibility limits for HUD's major assistance programs. Unlike poverty thresholds, relative income thresholds vary across the country.[7] These thresholds are based on reported household income, the number of people in the household, and geographic location.[8] In all but two age groups, the share of renters with incomes below 50 percent of median exceeds the share of renters with incomes above 95 percent of median.[9] Elderly renters are far more likely to have incomes below 50 percent of median and far less likely to have incomes above 95 percent of median than are non-elderly renters. Seventy percent of elderly renters have incomes below 50 percent of median compared to 36 percent of younger renters, reflecting the fact that those in better economic circumstances are very likely to have become homeowners by the time they reach age 65.

The preceding tables showed that the oldest and youngest age groups have the highest poverty rates and that those under age 18 are more likely to be poor than are the elderly. This observation, combined with recent divergent trends in the poverty rates of children and the elderly, gives rise to concern by some that the elderly are benefitting at the expense of children. However, a review of poverty rates since 1939 shows dramatic reductions in poverty rates for both groups.[10] Poverty rates among the elderly decreased from almost 78 percent in 1939 to 25.3 percent by 1969. Poverty rates for children under age 15 were estimated at 79.5 percent in 1939, dropping to 14.0 percent (for those under age 18) by 1969. Since then, elderly poverty rates have continued to decline (to 9.7 percent in 1999) while child poverty rates rose until about 1993, declining since then to 16.9 percent in 1999. Although government policy contributed significantly to the decline in poverty among the elderly in the last several decades, the disappointing trend in the earnings of the parents of children, not government policy *per se*, was primarily responsible for rising poverty among children.

Persistence of Poverty

The official measure of poverty considers the number of households who are poor in a single year. Since households may be poor for longer or shorter periods than one year, the time period used in measuring poverty affects the share of the population classified as poor. Households that are persistently poor may face greater need than those who experience only transitory poverty since the latter may be able to draw on other resources to meet their consumption needs.

Although poverty has typically been measured based on annual income, eligibility for major U.S. assistance programs is based on monthly rather than annual income. Ruggles (1990) and Ruggles and Williams (1987) used data from the Survey of Income and Program Participation (SIPP) to look at short term poverty spells. As Table 3 demonstrates, a much higher fraction of people were poor in at least one month than were poor all 12 months.[11] Although the share of elderly who were poor in any month was lower than the average for all persons, nearly 37 percent of elderly who were poor in at least one month were poor in all 12 months, compared to 23 percent of the entire population. Single parents with children constituted the only group with a higher share that was poor all 12 months (42.7 percent of those who were poor in at least one month).

Ruggles (1990) also showed that although fewer elderly have a poverty entrance, the share of the elderly who are still poor in any month exceeds that of the total population and that of children. Using 32 months of data from the 1984 SIPP panel, and defining 1/12 of the annual poverty threshold as the monthly poverty threshold, she found that 12.9 percent of those over age 65 entered poverty compared to 25.1 percent of the total sample. However, only 6.6 percent of all poverty spells lasted 24 months or more, compared to 16.7 percent of elderly poverty spells. For those under age 18, 32.5 percent entered poverty during the sample period, and 6.5 percent of their poverty spells lasted 24 months or more.[12]

TABLE 3. Poverty Rates (in Percent)
Computed from the 1984 Survey of Income and Program Participation

Family Type[a]	(1) Poor All 12 Months	(2) Poor in Any Month	(3) Col (1)/ Col (2)
All persons	5.9	26.2	22.5
Married couples with children	2.8	24.3	11.5
Single parents with children	25.8	60.8	42.4
Unrelated individuals	11.0	35.9	30.6
Other persons	2.0	14.3	14.0
Elderly persons[b]	6.8	18.5	36.8

[a] Persons are classified by family type, but poverty rates are reported for individuals.

[b] Elderly persons are aged 65 and over. They are also included in the previous 4 categories.

Source: Ruggles (1990), Table 5.1

A number of studies using data from the late 1960s through the 1970s found that the elderly were a disproportionate share of the persistently poor. When data were tabulated separately for households headed by elderly men and women, persons living in households headed by elderly women were more likely to experience persistent poverty than those in households headed by elderly men. Table 4 summarizes the results of this research. Because the authors of these studies employed several different definitions of persistent poverty and the studies covered different time periods, rates of persistent poverty varied. Although about 13 percent of the population lived in households headed by an elderly person in 1978 (Duncan, Coe, and Hill, 1984), persons living in elderly households comprised 22 to 36 percent of those in persistent poverty. The studies by Coe (1978) and Hill (1981) which defined persistent poverty as poor in all years found the elderly to be a smaller share of the persistently poor (22 to 26 percent) than did the other studies. This was most evident in the paper by Hill (1981) which included two different definitions of persistent poverty. The elderly accounted for 26 percent of the persistently poor

TABLE 4. Elderly Share of the Persistently Poor

Author(s)	Years of Data (PSID)	Definition of Persistently Poor	Share of Persistently Poor Persons In Households Headed by an Elderly:		
			Person	Woman	Man
Levy (1977)	1967-75	In poverty (Census poverty thresholds) at least 5 years between 1967 and 1973.	22.6%	not avail.	not avail.
Coe (1978)	1967-75	In poverty (Census poverty thresholds) every year from 1967 through 1975.	22.1%	not avail.	not avail.
Hill (1981)	1969-78	In poverty (Census poverty thresholds) at least 8 out of 10 years.	32.4%	17.5%	14.9%
		In poverty (Census poverty thresholds) every year from 1969 through 1978.	26.4%	22.2%	4.2%
Rainwater (1981)	1967-76	Always in poverty (relative income definition–below 50% of median) over 3 income averaging periods, 1967-76.	35.7%[a]	not avail.	not avail.
Duncan, Coe, Hill (1984)	1969-78	In poverty (Census poverty thresholds) 8 or more years.	33.0%	18.0%	15.0%

[a] Data for white non-Hispanic households only.

Sources: Ruggles (1990), Tables 5.7 and 5.8; Levy (1977) Table 9; Coe (1978) Table 8.2; Hill (1981) Table 3.5; Rainwater (1981) Table 3; and Duncan, Coe, and Hill (1984) Table 2.2.

when only those who were poor in every year were included, but 32 percent when only 8 of 10 years were required.[13]

Newman and Struyk (1984) used data from the Panel Study of Income Dynamics (PSID) for 1974 through 1978 and found that over 80 percent of the elderly who were poor in 1974 remained poor in at least 3 of the next 5 years compared to 51 percent for all heads of households who were poor in 1974. Their results also showed that those in female-headed elderly households were more likely to remain poor than were those in male-headed elderly households. Elderly blacks were slightly more likely to be classified as permanently poor than were persons in elderly white households.

In a more recent study, Burkhauser, Duncan, and Hauser (1994) employed PSID income data for 1983 through 1988 to compare the economic well-being of different age groups. In contrast to the studies discussed above, they used relative income measures–based on 50 percent and 40 percent of national median income–to compare the percentage of people in persistent poverty. An individual was considered to be persistently poor if the individual belonged to a family whose permanent income, defined as the family's average income over the six year period, adjusted for family size, was below 40 or 50 percent of the median permanent income. The youngest and oldest age groups were most likely to be persistently poor. Using a poverty threshold equal to 50 percent of national median income, one-quarter of those under age 10 or over 65 in 1983 were persistently poor, compared to 16 percent of the entire population. Reducing the poverty threshold to 40 percent of median income decreased the overall rate of persistent poverty from 16.1 to 10.2 percent. However, the age patterns remained much the same. The oldest and youngest groups were over 50 percent more likely to be persistently poor than was the population as a whole. Females were far more likely than males to be persistently poor; the overall rate of persistent poverty was 35 percent higher for females than males.

Burkhauser, Duncan, and Hauser also compared incomes with and without government assistance to illustrate the effect of government policies on persistent poverty. The data cited above reflect "after government" income which consists of family income plus government transfers net of personal taxes and social security contributions.[14] Clearly, Social Security and other programs have improved the well-being of the elderly. The overall rate of persistent poverty was 22.1 percent before government transfers and 16.1 percent after. Comparable rates for the elderly were 57.7 percent and 24.5 percent, respectively. Children benefitted less from government transfers. Their poverty rate only declined from 26.8 percent before to 24.8 percent after government transfers.

Asset Holdings of the Elderly

Income alone does not provide a complete picture of household well-being because it excludes wealth. Household wealth can provide a source of income through interest, rents, or, dividends; be drawn down in retirement to supplement other sources of income; yield consumption benefits not often captured in measures of money income (e.g., housing); and provide a form of insurance which can be used in times of need. Because income is not level across one's lifetime, wealth and borrowing provide a way to stabilize consumption patterns. Young households may borrow money to finance their education or to purchase a home. As households age, they tend to accumulate more wealth, which they may draw down in retirement. Therefore, the amount of wealth held at different ages is expected to vary.

When wealth is considered in addition to cash income, the economic status of the aged improves relative to that of younger households. Table 5 compares the level and distribution of household net worth for the elderly and all households using data from the Survey of Income and Program Participation (SIPP) reported in Radner (1989). The median net worth of elderly households in 1984 exceeded that of younger households as a group. Median net worth was highest for householders aged 55 to 64, $72,460 (not shown), and next highest for those aged 65 to 74, $62,060. The higher net worth of households in the 55 to 64 age group reflects the fact that this cohort (born between 1920 and 1929) earned more during their peak earning years than their predecessors and the fact that many were still saving rather than dis-saving.

Although the elderly as a group had a higher median net worth than households under age 65, the data in Table 5 also show a great deal of variation in the distribution of wealth holding, both within and across age groups. Thirty per-

TABLE 5. Percentage Distribution of Households by Net Worth and Age of Householder,1984

Net Worth	All Ages	Aged 65 or older		
		All	65-74	75 or older
Number of households (in millions)	86.9	18.2	10.7	7.5
Median Net Worth	$32,600	$59,680	$62,060	$54,620
Percent Distribution				
Negative or $0	11	7	7	6
$1-9,999	21	13	11	15
$10,000-$24,999	12	9	9	10
$25,000-$49,999	15	16	15	17
$50,000-$99,999	20	26	26	25
$100,000-$249,999	16	24	25	23
$250,000 or more	4	6	7	4
Percent < $25,000	44	29	27	31

Source: Radner (1989), Table 1.

cent of elderly households reported their net worth at $100,000 or more, while a similar share, 29 percent, had wealth of less than $25,000. Twenty percent of elderly households reported net worth of less than $10,000. Among all households, only 20 percent had assets of $100,000 or more, and 44 percent reported a net worth of less than $25,000.

A fuller picture of economic well-being appears when income and wealth holding are considered together. Radner (1989) looked at the joint distribution of households with relatively low income and relatively low net worth.[15] Not surprisingly, a sizeable share of young households, one-quarter of those under age 25, reported both low income and low net worth. Compared with households aged 35 to 64, a larger share of elderly households had both low income and low net worth.[16]

HOUSING PROBLEMS AMONG ELDERLY RENTERS

In programs like Supplemental Security Income (SSI) and Temporary Assistance to Needy Families (TANF), all families who meet the eligibility criteria are entitled to receive benefits. This is not true of housing assistance programs. Low-income families and elderly households (those with incomes below 80 percent of the adjusted median income for their area) are eligible for benefits, but there is insufficient funding to provide housing assistance for everyone. In this section, we use American Housing Survey (AHS) data to consider the housing problems faced by households of different ages and the extent of housing assistance received by different groups.[17] Since there are notable differences in income among different age groups of the elderly, detailed age groups are reported when the sample size permits.

Incidence of Housing Problems

There are a variety of ways of measuring the housing problems faced by households. Here we employ a summary indicator which measures the share of households with one or more of three problems: excessive cost burden, physical inadequacy, or overcrowding.[18] In accord with the guidelines used in many federal housing programs, households paying more than 30 percent of their income for housing are considered to be paying an excess cost burden. Physically inadequate units are those classified in the American Housing Survey as either moderately or severely inadequate.[19] Households are considered overcrowded when there is more than one person per room. To measure the age of the household, we use the age of the reference person, assumed here to be the "head of household."[20]

Although this study focuses on renters, it seems helpful to contrast them with owners. The homeownership rate is 64 percent for all households compared to 77 percent for elderly households. In contrast, only 14 percent of households headed by a person under age 25 and 44 percent of households headed by a person between age 25 and 34 are homeowners (Table 6). Homeownership rates are highest among those aged 65 to 69–82 percent–and next highest among those aged 70 to 74–80 percent. The homeownership rate is slightly lower, 73 percent, among those over age 74.

Renters of all ages face more housing problems than owners, and older renters experience problems more often than younger households. Table 6 shows the share of households of different tenure and age groups experiencing one or

TABLE 6. Housing Characteristics by Age of Head of Household

				Age of Head of Household			
	All Ages	Under 25	25 to 34	35 to 44	45 to 64	65 to 69	70 to 74	75 and over
Homeownership Rate	64.2%	14.3%	43.9%	65.7%	77.1%	81.8%	79.8%	72.7%
Share of Households with One or More Housing Problems								
Renters	48.3	53.9	42.0	43.8	48.7	63.3	66.3	66.9
Owners	23.6	33.9	25.5	23.8	20.0	25.4	24.9	29.4
Share of Households Paying Over 30 Percent of Income for Housing								
Renters	41.2	49.8	34.5	33.8	41.0	59.0	60.6	64.3
Owners	18.5	28.5	19.6	18.1	15.6	20.3	19.9	23.7
Share of Renter Households:								
Paying Over 50% of Income for Housing	19.0	27.2	14.8	15.0	18.6	25.3	27.3	31.7
Overcrowded	4.9	3.6	6.1	7.4	4.1	1.0	.4	.4
Inadequate Housing	11.2	9.1	10.4	12.9	12.9	9.9	11.8	8.9
Very Low Income with Priority Problems	18.3	25.7	14.3	14.4	18.3	25.0	25.8	28.3

	All Ages	Under 25	25 to 34	35 to 44	45 to 64	65 to 74	75 and over
Receipt of Housing Assistance by Renters, 1989 (thousands of households)							
Total Assisted Renters	4,071	248	936	665	804	659	759
Income Eligible Renters[a]	13,808	1,516	3,866	2,298	2,551	1,634	1,943
Total Renter Households	33,768	3,552	12,406	6,845	6,191	2,364	2,410
Assisted/Income-Eligible	0.29	0.16	0.24	0.29	0.32	0.40	0.39
Income-Eligible/Total Renters	0.41	0.43	0.31	0.34	0.41	0.69	0.81

[a] Income-eligible renters are those who would qualify for admission to assisted housing on the basis of their reported income.

more housing problems. Among non-elderly renters, the share with problems ranges from 42 to 54 percent, but, among elderly renters, the share ranges from 63 percent for those aged 65 to 69 to over 66 percent for those over 70. Elderly owners fare about as well as younger owners. They face a slightly higher incidence of problems than those aged 35 to 64 but a lower share of problems than owners under age 25.

Among all age groups, the most common housing problem is affordability, and again, renters face problems more often than owners. Overall, 19 percent of owners face excess cost burdens, that is, pay more than 30 percent of their income for housing, compared to 41 percent of renters (Table 6). The oldest renters have a higher incidence of excess cost burdens than do younger renters. From 34 to 50 percent of non-elderly renters have excess cost burdens compared to 59 percent to 64 percent of elderly renters. Sixty-four percent of renters age 75 or older have excess cost burdens; this is a higher rate of affordability problems than any other age group. Within the non-elderly population, renter households under age 25 also experience a high rate of affordability problems; half of these households pay over 30 percent of their income for housing.

A smaller share of households face a more serious affordability problem, paying over half their income for housing. Table 6 shows that, as with excess cost burdens, the oldest households along with the youngest are the most likely to pay over half their income for rent. Among those over age 74, slightly less than one-third of renters pay severe cost burdens, compared to 15 to 19 percent of households aged 25 to 64.

Far fewer households of all ages experience one of the other two housing problems: overcrowding and physical inadequacy. Because most households headed by a person age 65 or older contain only one or two people, few elderly households are overcrowded. The overall share of overcrowded households is low, with the highest rate of 7.4 percent occurring in renter households in which head of the household is age 35 to 44 (Table 6). More renters live in inadequate rather than overcrowded units. Overall, 11 percent of renters lived in units that were either moderately or severely inadequate. The share of renters living in physically inadequate housing varies relatively little with age, ranging from about 9 to 13 percent.

The incidence of housing problems is strongly related to income. As Table 7 shows, the share of elderly households with one or more housing problems declines as income rises. About three-quarters of elderly households whose incomes are below 50 percent of local median income face one or more housing problems, and, as Table 2 showed, 70 percent of elderly renter households fall into this income category. The share of elderly households with housing problems is much lower among households whose incomes are above 80 percent of median.

In part due to their lower incomes, minority renters face more housing problems than do white non-Hispanic renters. In 1991, 43 percent of all white

TABLE 7. Share of Elderly Renter Households with One or More Housing Problems

Income Group (by share of median income)	Share with Problems
30% or less	76.9%
30-50%	74.8
50-80%	62.0
80-95%	26.6
Above 95%	16.8
Total	65.9

Source: Tabulations of the 1991 AHS by the authors.

non-Hispanic renters, 57 percent of black non-Hispanic renters, and 64 percent of Hispanic renters faced one or more housing problems.

Renter households whose incomes fall below 80 percent of the HUD-adjusted median family income for their area are income-eligible for housing assistance.[21] In previous years, federal preference rules gave priority for admission to those with very low incomes who occupied substandard housing, paid more than 50 percent of their income for rent, or were displaced.[21] Very low-income households with these priority problems have been described as those with "worst case" housing needs (U.S. Department of Housing and Urban Development, 1991).

Table 6 shows that the incidence of "worst case" housing needs is highest among the oldest and youngest renter households. Among those under 25 or over 64, the share of renters who are very low income and have priority problems ranges from 25 to 28 percent. In comparison, only 18 percent of all very low-income renters have worst case needs. Clearly, elderly renters and renters under age 25 experience worst case needs more often than renters in other age groups.

Participation in Housing Assistance Programs

A larger share of elderly than non-elderly renters were income-eligible for housing assistance in 1989. The bottom panel of Table 6 compares the number of renter households receiving housing assistance in 1989 with the number that were eligible for assistance based on their income. As the last row of the table illustrates, over two-thirds of renter households whose head was age 65 or older were eligible for housing assistance, compared to less than 43 percent of younger households. Among the oldest group, those aged 75 or older, 4 out of 5 renters were income-eligible for housing assistance.

The share of income-eligible households receiving assistance increased with age (Table 6). In 1989, only 16 percent of eligible households under age

25 received housing assistance compared with 24 to 34 percent of those aged 25 to 64 and around 40 percent of those aged 65 and over. A number of factors explain the higher share of elderly receiving housing assistance. First, even among the income-eligible, a greater fraction of the elderly has very low income. As Table 2 showed, elderly renters were almost twice as likely as non-elderly renters to have very low incomes. Second, since it may take a few years to move to the top of a housing assistance waiting list, households receiving assistance will be older than those on the waiting list. The waiting list *may* also screen out households with only short spells of poverty, concentrating assistance on groups, such as the elderly, which have higher than average rates of persistent poverty. Finally, the existence of the Section 202 program, which targets assistance to the elderly, undoubtedly raises the share of assistance going to the elderly.

CONCLUSION

When seeking answers to the problem of how to best utilize scarce housing assistance resources, policy makers must recognize that needs can vary tremendously even within traditional population classifications. Today it often makes little sense to speak broadly of the housing problems of families when the proper focus should be on, say, the problems of single-parent families with children. Similarly, when discussing the housing problems of the elderly, it is important that the elderly not be regarded as a homogeneous group when it is more meaningful to consider the problems of populations like elderly females over age 75 or the persistently poor elderly.

This article has shown that the overall improvement in the economic well-being of the elderly in recent times (as indicated by a falling poverty rate) masks the problems of certain sub-groups within the elderly population. The persistently poor and near poor elderly are two such groups. Although the elderly are less likely to experience a spell of poverty than those under age 65, a disproportionate share of the poor elderly is persistently poor. In addition, elderly persons are more likely than the overall population to be near poor. Within the elderly population, renters, female-headed, minority, and older elderly households tend to be worse off than others. Low-income households have a greater likelihood of living in housing that is unaffordable, inadequate, or overcrowded, and the elderly are no exception. As is true for most households, the housing problems of the elderly center on affordability. The high incidence of worst case needs among elderly renters is chiefly due to affordability problems stemming from low incomes.

Circumstances also vary tremendously within the remainder of the population. Within the non-elderly population, single-parent families with children, and young persons as a group, are among the worst off in terms of the incidence and persistence of poverty. These groups also account for a disproportionate share of those whose incomes are less than half the poverty line, and many have worst-case housing needs. As is true within the elderly population, female-headed and minority renter households tend to be worse off than others.

The data employed in much of this article are from the early part of the 1990s. The cohort of individuals who have reached age 65 in the past 10 years lived in better economic circumstances than the preceding birth cohort and thus are less likely to be poor than were earlier elderly individuals. This should not divert attention from the fact that many subgroups within the elderly population, such as renters, still face economic hardships, including housing affordability problems.

NOTES

1. In addition to Federal rental assistance, there are other programs which directly or indirectly provide housing assistance to low-income or disabled renter households. See Newman and Schnare (1988) and Newman and Schnare (1992). Newman and Schnare (1988) estimate that the welfare system spent about $10 billion on housing assistance in 1983.

2. According to this preference system, very low-income households (those whose incomes are less than 50 percent of the local median income, with adjustments for family size and local housing market conditions) who paid more than 50 percent of their income for rent, lived in substandard housing, or were involuntarily displaced would go to the top of waiting lists maintained by local public housing authorities. Now, local authorities can establish their own preferences.

3. The Appendix briefly describes several issues related to the measurement of poverty, including the establishment of poverty thresholds.

4. In some parts of this article, households, rather than families, will be the unit of analysis. A household includes all persons sharing a housing unit, while a family is defined by the Census Bureau as persons living in the same household who are related to the householder by birth, marriage, or adoption. In many cases a family and a household are the same. Under the Census Bureau definition, individuals living alone are not considered to be a family.

5. Income data for 1990 as reported in the March 1991 Current Population Survey.

6. Poverty thresholds for families were applied to households to obtain household poverty rates.

7. For a family of 4, the thresholds used to create Table 2 varied from about 93 percent to 256 percent of the average poverty threshold weighted to reflect household composition.

8. Income limits are set for metropolitan areas and non-metropolitan counties as identified in the American Housing Survey (AHS). Income thresholds for smaller metropolitan areas and all non-metropolitan areas are based on averages for broader geographic areas in the same Census region.

9. Because the medians used to compute the thresholds include owners as well as renters, it is not surprising that less than one-third of renters report incomes above 95 percent of median. In addition, the adjustments for local housing costs and other factors mean that in some places less than half of all households (owners and renters) have incomes above the median.

10. The poverty rates cited here are from Smolensky et. al (1988), using decennial Census data, and Dalaker and Proctor (2000), using the Current Population Survey.

11. Although the table reports family composition, it shows the share of *persons* in poverty. For example, the second line of the table shows that 2.8 percent of persons in families consisting of married couples with children were poor in all twelve months.

12. Ruggles found similar results using two alternative definitions of poverty to eliminate short poverty spells that result from very small fluctuations in income. See Ruggles (1990).

13. Interestingly, the composition of the elderly poor differed dramatically under these two definitions. When only those who were poor in all years were counted as persistently poor, persons in households headed by an elderly woman constituted a larger share and persons in households headed by an elderly man constituted a smaller share of the persistently poor compared to the less stringent 8 of 10 years definition of persistence.

14. Both measures of income include the in-cash value of food stamps and the imputed rental value of owner-occupied housing. To adjust the relative income thresholds for family size, the authors employed the family size equivalence scale implicit in the U.S. poverty thresholds.

15. Relatively low income is defined as the bottom quintile of the income distribution for all ages, and relatively low net worth is defined as the bottom two quintiles of the distribution of net worth for all ages, adjusting both for household size.

16. Radner found similar results using financial assets rather than net worth as a measure of wealth.

17. The American Housing Survey (AHS) contains a substantial amount of information about U.S. households and their housing conditions. The AHS is a sample survey of household and housing unit characteristics conducted by the Census Bureau for HUD. The AHS refers to two surveys, a national survey, conducted every other year, and a set of metropolitan surveys. The data tabulations included here were produced from the 1991 National file of the AHS.

18. This measure or similar measures are frequently used in housing policy work. For example, see Bogdon, Silver, and Turner (1993).

19. As reported in Newman and Schnare (1993), severely inadequate units are those which: (a) lack basic systems such as plumbing or electricity; (b) have nonfunctioning systems such as plumbing, heating, or electricity; (c) have five of six maintenance problems (leaks from outdoors, leaks from indoors, holes in the floor, holes or open cracks in the walls or ceilings, more than a square foot of peeling paint or plaster, or rats in the past 90 days); or (d) have all four problems in public areas (no working light fixtures; loose or missing steps; loose or missing railings; and no elevator). Moderately inadequate units are those which are not severely inadequate, but have one or more of the following problems: (a) all toilets broken down simultaneously, at least three times in the prior three months for at least six hours each time; (b) unvented heating systems; (c) any three of the six severe maintenance problems listed under severe inadequacy; (d) any three of the four severe public area problems noted above; or (e) lack a complete kitchen (a sink, range, and refrigerator available for the exclusive use of the occupants of the unit).

20. For ease of exposition, the term "head of household" is used to refer to the reference person. In the case of a married couple household, the reference person can be either spouse. When the household consists only of unrelated individuals, the reference person is the person (or one of the people) in whose name the unit is rented.

21. Families and elderly or handicapped single persons are eligible for assistance. Single persons below age 62 who are not disabled are eligible only if there are not enough other applicants for assistance.

22. Local housing authorities can now set their own priorities for assistance within the general income guidelines.

23. The brief discussion here highlights some issues to consider when comparing incomes or poverty rates. For a more complete discussion, see Palmer, Smeeding, and Jencks (1988) and Ruggles (1990).

24. When the insurance value of Medicare benefits is included in elderly income, their poverty rate declines markedly. However, as Radner (1992) notes, medical needs are higher among the elderly than among the younger population.

REFERENCES

Bogdon, Amy S., Joshua Silver, and Margery Austin Turner. 1993. *National Analysis of Housing Affordability, Adequacy, and Availability: A Framework for Local Housing Strategies.* Report prepared for the U.S. Department of Housing and Urban Development. The Urban Institute, Washington, DC, May.

Burkhauser, Richard V., Greg J. Duncan, and Richard Hauser. 1994. Sharing Prosperity Across the Age Distribution: A Comparison of the United States and Germany in the 1980s. *The Gerontologist,* 34 (2): 150-160.

Casey, Connie H. 1992. *Characteristics of HUD-Assisted Renters and Their Units in 1989.* Washington, DC: Office of Policy Development and Research, U.S. Department of Housing and Urban Development, March.

Coe, Richard. 1978. Dependency and Poverty in the Short Run, in *Five Thousand Families–Patterns of Economic Progress,* Vol. VI, pp. 273-296.

Dalaker, Joseph, and Bernadette D. Proctor. 2000. *Poverty in the United States: 1999.* Washington, DC: U.S. Government Printing Office, Current Population Reports, Series P60-210.

Duncan, Greg J., Richard D. Coe, and Martha S. Hill. 1984. The Dynamics of Poverty, in Greg J. Duncan (ed.) *Years of Poverty, Years of Plenty,* Institute for Social Research, Ann Arbor, pp. 33-69.

Hill, Martha S. 1981. Some Dynamic Aspects of Poverty, in *Five Thousand Families–Patterns of Economic Progress,* Vol. IX, pp. 93-120.

Levy, Frank. 1977. How Big is the American Underclass? Urban Institute Working Paper 00090-1. The Urban Institute, Washington, DC.

Newman, Sandra J., and Ann B. Schnare.1988. *Beyond Bricks and Mortar: Reexamining the Purpose and Effects of Housing Assistance,* The Urban Institute, Washington, DC.

_____ 1993. Last in Line: Housing Assistance for Households with Children. *Housing Policy Debate,* 4 (3): 417-455.

_____ 1992. *Subsidizing Shelter: The Relationship Between Welfare and Housing Assistance,* The Urban Institute, Washington, DC.

Newman, Sandra J., and Raymond J. Struyk. 1984. An Alternative Targeting Strategy for Housing Assistance. *The Gerontologist,* 24 (6): 584-592.

Palmer, John L., Timothy Smeeding, and Christopher Jencks. 1988. The Uses and Limits of Income Comparisons, in Palmer, Smeeding, and Torrey (eds.) *The Vulnerable,* The Urban Institute, Washington, DC.

Radner, Daniel B. 1992. The Economic Status of the Aged. *Social Security Bulletin,* Fall, 55 (3): 3-23.

_____ 1989. Net Worth and Financial Assets of Age Groups in 1984. *Social Security Bulletin,* March, 52 (3): 2-15.

Rainwater, Lee. 1981. Persistent and Transitory Poverty: A New Look. Working Paper No. 70. Joint Center for Urban Studies of MIT and Harvard, Cambridge, MA.

Ruggles, Patricia. 1990. *Drawing the Line: Alternative Poverty Measures and Their Implications for Policy.* The Urban Institute, Washington, DC.

Ruggles, Patricia, and Roberton Williams. 1987. Transitions In and Out of Poverty: New Data from the Survey of Income and Program Participation. SIPP Working Paper 8716, December.

Smolensky, Eugene, Sheldon Danziger, and Peter Gottschalk. 1988. The Declining Significance of Age in the United States: Trends in the Well-Being of Children and the Elderly since 1939, in Palmer, Smeeding, and Torrey (eds.) *The Vulnerable,* The Urban Institute, Washington, DC.

U.S. Bureau of the Census. 1991. *Poverty in the United States: 1990.* Current Population Reports, Series P-60, No. 175. Washington, DC: U.S. Government Printing Office.

U.S. Department of Housing and Urban Development, Office of Policy Development and Research 1991. *Priority Problems and "Worst Case" Needs in 1989: A Report to Congress.*

APPENDIX–MEASURING POVERTY

Ideally, we would like to compare the well-being of different groups of individuals and households. However, since many intangible factors affect well-being, to make the problem more tractable we must limit the investigation to measurable criteria, that is, material or economic well-being.[23] The discussion in this article focuses chiefly on income measures of well-being and compares poverty rates among the elderly and other groups.

Money income provides a useful measure of the material well-being of different groups and, along with absolute or relative measures of poverty, is often used to compare different groups. Data on money income are readily available to researchers through numerous surveys, some of which follow the same individuals over time. In addition, income can be compared across and within demographic groups and can be disaggregated by source.

The disadvantage of using income to compare different groups is that our ultimate interest is in economic well-being (or consumption), which is influenced by many factors other than current income. Other types of economic resources, such as wealth, insurance, and in-kind transfers, are not captured in current income measures. In addition, to compare different groups, income must be adjusted to reflect demographic characteristics. That is, we need some way to adjust measures of household income to reflect household size and the varying needs of household members of different ages.

We can compare the economic well-being of individuals and households using absolute or relative standards. Absolute standards define poverty as income below some absolute measure that represents an "objective" minimum. The advantage of using an absolute standard is that it provides a fixed benchmark that can be used to measure progress in reducing poverty over time. However, its disadvantage is that it is difficult to establish an "objective" minimum that is applicable over a long period or across divergent population groups. Official poverty rate statistics are based on an absolute standard established in the late 1960s, updated annually for inflation.

Relative measures of poverty compare income or consumption to social norms of some type, which change. Among the most common relative measures are those which establish cutoffs that are some fraction of local or national median income. For example, eligibility for many HUD programs is based on a relative income standard, which varies across metropolitan areas and non-metropolitan counties. A disadvantage of using a relative measure is that it presents a "moving target" against which to judge anti-poverty policy.

The poverty measure used in official statistics is derived from work by Orshansky in the 1960s. She first estimated food budgets for families of different size and composition, using data from the Department of Agriculture. Based on a USDA study which estimated food costs as one-third of a family's total budget, she multiplied the food budget by 3 to arrive at total budgets. The Orshansky measure of poverty for a family of four was approximately half of national median income when it was introduced, but by the 1990s was only about one-third of median income.

The official poverty thresholds used by the federal government are lower for the elderly than for those under age 65. The elderly are assumed to need less food, so the starting point for computing the poverty line is lower. However, using a constant multiplier of three to compute the poverty line from the food budget assumes that the elderly's expenses for other items, such as housing and medical care, are also commensurately lower than for younger households. While this may underestimate the number of poor older persons living in poverty, the exclusion of the value of Medicare benefits may cause the poverty rate for the elderly to be overstated.[24]

Money income is the basis for measuring poverty in official government statistics. Income is measured before payment of personal income taxes, Social Security taxes, dues, etc. Therefore, money income does not reflect the fact that some families receive part of their income in the form of in-kind benefits, such as food stamps, health benefits, or subsidized housing.

Index